I0095301

MOON BLOOD

AVIVA

Copyright © 2023 by Aviva
All rights reserved. No part of this book may be used, reproduced, stored in a retrieval system, or transmitted in any form or by any means – electronic, mechanical, photocopy, recording, scanning or other – except for brief quotes in critical reviews or articles without the prior written permission from the publisher.

CyclicalHealing.com

ISBN: 979-8-9891597-0-3

Editor, Book Cover and Interior Design:
Micah Schwader
www.inspiredlifepublications.com

Cover Art & Pointillism Drawings:
Andres Villalon
@verdeser.art

Paintings: Eduardo Paras
@eduparas_arte

Acknowledgments

I am full of gratitude for all of the magical beings who have supported the creation of this book.

Years ago, Kristen Damato supported me in gaining clarity about my visions, and it was then that I began to nurture two special seeds, one of which became *Moon Blood*, another of which became my first original medicine music album *Memoria Ancestral*.

To my editor, publisher, and mentor, Micah Schwader, who helped me bring this project to completion and to discover along the way that this book is only the beginning of a continuously unfolding cyclical healing journey. Micah has helped me to create a platform where I can step fully into my service of creative expression, womb work, storytelling, and inspiring others to connect to their authentic medicine. He has been present for me throughout the fear, the doubts, the joy, and the celebrations. He continues to be a consistent presence, accompanying me to birth this book.

To all of the places I have called home throughout this writing process. Each in its way has provided a temple space for me to work on my laptop while also being deeply immersed in the mountains. Thank you, Gaiatree Sanctuary in Northern California, Karuna Community in Lake Atitlan, and Vilcabamba, Ecuador. Although much of the story and wisdom poured into this book has been compiled over many years, most of the writing took place in these locations—my homes, my bases, and extensions of my body merging with the land.

To the wise medicine women who generously shared their life experiences and sacred ancestral teachings. Thank you for recognizing and honoring the medicine that I carry.

To my mom for always supporting me to follow my intuition and create my own life path. I know it is scary and vulnerable for your daughter to share such intimate life stories with the world. Thank you for understanding that writing and publishing this book is integral to my healing journey. Thank you for instilling the courage, strength, and determination to follow my dreams. Your hard-working, compassionate, loving heart is a source of inspiration for me. Thank you for showing up in service to support so many people, for your commitment toward personal growth, and for bringing me on to this Earth to continue your legacy with my own flavor.

To all the lovers, crushes, and sexual partners who have danced into my life. I have learned so much about myself through your medicine, which was, at times, sweet and, at other times, bitter. But know that it was always medicine to heal through your reflection.

To my dad for being a father in the best way he knew. Thank you for being a part of bringing me onto this Earth and teaching me forgiveness, acceptance, and compassion.

To all guardian angels and light beings who accompany and guide my journey.

To the rivers that have restored me, the sweet smokes of incense that have cleansed me, the grandfather fire who has helped me to release and transform, and to the Pachamama for her infinite abundance.

To the moon, for being a constant source of inspiration through her shadow and light, reflecting our cyclical nature.

To the master plants who have deepened my connection to my intuition and the natural world and have reminded me how to love.

To all of the embodiment practices that have supported me in integrating my healing into my cellular memory. Specifically

What People Are Saying About Moon Blood

"Through compelling storytelling, Aviva's words quench an ancient thirst. *Moon Blood* provides us the opportunity to experience healing through a remembering of our interconnectedness with the Earth, the Moon, our bodies, and each other as we reawaken to the wisdom that pours through when we align with the rhythms of our cycles."

~ Kristen D'Amato,
author of *We Choose Love: Redefining Our Relationship to Healing - An Empowering Approach to Chronic Conditions & Beyond*

"*Moon Blood* is a powerful book about a deeply personal healing journey. Aviva's travels and encounters are fuel for learning more about her body and her power, and we are so fortunate to learn from them! This book has practical tools for engaging in a deeper relationship with your womb and menstruation journey. Aviva acknowledges the difficulties and nuances of this process while supporting us throughout the journey and reminding us of our shared humanity. She also includes useful tips for nutrition, movement, and rest, while encouraging readers to listen to their own bodies first and foremost. So powerful and transformative!'"

~ Alison R., Kundalini Yoga Instructor and Activist

"Aviva's *Moon Blood* takes the reader through a wondrous trail of discovery of the feminine menstrual blood mysteries. The reader is guided through ancient traditional practices, personal revelations, archetypal and astrological parallels, and true stories that form a cohesive account of healing from sexual trauma. Aviva's book is a travelogue through both South America and her psyche, ready to be healed using the ancient tool of being in complete sync with one's changing moon cycles and, through that, with Mother Nature."

~ Eostar, Singer-songwriter and Medicine Woman

"Moon Blood offers a reflection and an invitation for me to continue to deepen and expand my relationship to all my cycles, my body as an Earth altar, and the wholeness of my being in interconnection to all of life."

~ Naya, Death & Birth Doula

"I wish I could gift this book to my thirteen-year-old self so that she could accept the nature of her cycle, understand the apothecary of plants around her, and love herself and her partners better. Even at 31, *Moon Blood* has helped me do all these things."

~ Katie Rose Criscuolo, Songstress

"In her gripping account of her healing journey, Aviva skillfully explores the complexities of holding deep compassion for herself alongside compassion for everyone she encounters — even through sexual trauma and heartache. Her stories beautifully capture the powerful intersections of tenderness meeting honesty, understanding meeting accountability, and magic meeting groundedness. Her capacity for nuanced, holistic self-reflection makes *Moon Blood* a moving invitation for discovery and healing."

~ Rosalee, Early Childhood Educator

the Contact Improvisation community of Argentina and the hula-hooping community all over South America.

To the voice practices that have led me to understand how we each carry medicine in our voice and our song carries the vibration we need to heal. Maryn Azoff, my vocal activation mentor, continues to inspire me with her creativity and dedication toward service for the good of all beings.

Thank you to my dear Chilean brother Andres Villalon for creating original illustrations for this book as well as redesigning the mandala for the *Moon Blood Journal* with endless patience and inspiration.

Thank you, Edu Paras, for creating original illustrations for each original song of my album *Memoria Ancestral*. A handful of these images appear perfectly in this book.

Thank you, readers, for witnessing my journey.

Content Warning

Throughout this book, you will come across several personal narratives that detail events such as sexual assault, womb trauma, and erotic snippets.

Writing these stories has supported my healing journey, and I invite you to dive into these experiences with me. You may be triggered at certain moments, and I believe that our triggers help us see what wounds within us are asking to be acknowledged and loved.

Please seek support from a trusted friend or mentor if any significant memories or emotions arise for you upon reading, and remember that you are not alone. I include this content warning to prepare and encourage you to be fully present throughout the journey, including the uncomfortable bits. Deep healing may emerge from the parts of these narratives that are most challenging.

Instead of shutting out the darkness, I invite you to get curious about your shadows and the stories of pain that may linger within you. If you want to share your personal experience upon reading and desire any individual support, you can contact me through cyclicalhealing.com.

With love,

Aviva

Content

Introduction

Moon Blood is an invitation to embark on a cyclical womb healing journey beginning with the dark phases of the waning and new moon and culminating in the luminous phases of the waxing and full moon. Through guided rituals, moon wisdom, and storytelling, you will deepen your connection to the elements of nature, the magic of your womb, your shadows, and your light. To accompany your cyclical journey, use the *Moon Blood: Cyclical Mandala Calendar* to begin tracking your cycles for thirteen moon cycles. This calendar is designed for all humans, regardless of whether you bleed monthly. As you listen deeply to your self through the passing of many moons, you will discover a wisdom so pure and unique that no one or nothing can teach you; she only comes from within.

~

In June 2017, at age twenty-two, I hopped on a plane with a one-way ticket to *El Caribe Colombiano*, the Colombian Caribbean. I began this journey with a Mirena IUD, an intrauterine plastic hormonal birth control device inserted in my womb.

I hadn't had a period in three years.

I had absolutely no connection to my menstrual cycle.

As I began meeting fierce women healers, they taught me about *La Luna*, referring to both the moon's cyclical relationship to the Earth and every bleeding person's cyclical relationship to their menstrual cycle. These inspiring women planted a seed of desire within me to heal my womb space, and they encouraged and supported me to discover the magical beauty of my cyclical being.

At first, I felt fear and resistance toward diving back into menstruation. I had previously loved that my "annoying period" had gone away for years. My entire socialization had centered on the narrative that periods were bothersome, gross, disgusting, shameful, and secretive. At the same time, I felt excited about this invitation for my moon time to be an opportunity to dive into self-care, ritual, magic, and honoring my body.

When I turned eighteen and began having sex with my first boyfriend, I started taking pharmaceutical birth control pills. For years, I continued taking some form of hormonal contraceptives even through long seasons in which I was not sexually active. Taking the pill seemed like the only "safe sex" option when I began exploring penetrative sex.

I lived in Israel for a year after graduating high school, and I remember taking a long bus ride to a distant clinic to see a gynecologist who would prescribe me the pill. I felt extremely nervous and begged my boyfriend to accompany me. After all, I was going through this whole process of putting hormones in my body so that we could have "safe sex." He refused to come with me. He said that his father never went to a gynecologist and that he would never go to a gynecologist. I insisted he didn't have to come inside, but he could at least take the bus with me and wait in the waiting room. He refused. He seemed embarrassed even to be having this conversation.

So, I took it upon myself to take the pill for one year. I experienced weight gain, mood swings, and extreme irritability throughout the year. I felt unsafe within my body, yet I never considered stopping the pill. When I arrived home to California, my doctor prescribed me a different pill that I tried for a few months, making everything much worse. The imbalances I felt within my emotional and physical body intensified. Eventually, my doctor suggested that I get an IUD. I agreed.

Years later, simply considering removing my IUD sent me on a profound emotional rollercoaster. I created space to feel sensations that were radically new and enticing and feel into deep fear. I noticed my protective mechanisms merging with societal fears in a fight against removing something from my body that had been serving as a contraceptive. Additionally, I had experienced a handful of sexual assaults in which men ejaculated inside of my body without my consent, and my IUD created a sense of safety and protection for me. Eventually, in divine timing, one experience at a permaculture community in Colombia finally led me to remove my IUD.

Mainly, single mothers and their children stewarded this community. There was so much beauty in how these women grew their food, created a mountain school for their children, and built their homes out of clay and bamboo. They lived in a unique ecosystem, a humid cloud forest with big trees and moist air, high up in the mountainous jungle, home to an incredible freezing river that flowed through the land.

I had exchanged emails with a woman who had provided me with basic directions on how to get to their small community farm in the mountains. She insisted that I do my best to arrive during the day because I could get lost in the forest at night. Since I had been hitchhiking that day, I felt that time was out of my control. Yet, I was doing my best to arrive with daylight. I finally arrived at an intersection on the outskirts of a small town where I could take a tiny bus to an even tinier town that would lead me to this community.

Unfortunately, by the time I arrived, the last bus was rolling through, and it was fully packed. I pleaded with the bus driver to make extra space for me and told him I was willing to curl up and sit on the floor. It felt essential that I take this bus so I did not have to stay in this random town overnight. The bus driver seemed resistant to the idea, but luckily, all the people on the bus heard what was going on, and they began cheering for me and insisting that he make space. The whole scene was hilarious, silly, and light-hearted. Ultimately, the bus driver gave in, and I sat on the floor for an extremely bumpy hour-long bus ride through which I answered endless questions about my travels and shared stories with the curious locals. When we arrived at the town, it was already getting dark, and inevitably, it began to rain. I felt hopeful because there was still a little light and the rain was not too heavy, and if everything went according to plan, I would only need to walk thirty minutes into the forest to arrive at the community.

The first directions led me to find train tracks and follow them toward the East. So, I oriented myself and began walking. As it got darker and started raining harder, seeing through the thick trees and cloud-filled skies became impossible. I had to move slowly to navigate my way through this wet, unknown jungle.

The directions indicated that I would need to cross two bridges. I was told that the first bridge I could cross with no problem. However, I could not cross over the second bridge and needed to find a trail underneath off to the side. She insisted I take this detoured trail to cross over the rushing river. After crossing the first bridge, I kept walking and heard the sound of a large roaring river. Although I could not see more than just a few feet ahead of what my flashlight could illuminate, my intuition told me I must be nearing the second bridge. I saw a large stretch of train tracks with big cracks and gaps between each piece of rotting wood. There was no way to cross this bridge, so I searched for the safer detoured side trail. I wandered off to the side in various attempts to locate this underpass, but I had no luck.

It was super dark.

I was soaking wet.

And I really wanted to arrive.

I contemplated pitching my tent and accepting my defeat and inability to cross the river. But somehow, I thought crossing the railroad-tracked ancient bridge would be a good idea. I took one step, and my legs began shaking uncontrollably. I peered over to see the rapids 100 feet below me, ravishing everything in its path at full speed. I felt there was no way to cross this bridge safely, and I considered taking a step back. But instead, I took a step forward. My most courageous, perhaps riskiest self kicked in at that moment and said, "Hey, you better stop shaking because you can easily slip off this bridge and be swallowed by the river. You must focus and center yourself in your breath to get to the other side alive."

I began to take deep breaths, and with each exhale, I reached one leg over the gap toward the next wooden plank of the train track. There were probably two-foot wide gaps between each plank, but each step felt like a two-mile leap. It's just like slacklining, I told myself, one step at a time. About one-quarter of the way across, my body was physically exhausted. Keeping my balance on the wet, slippery tracks as the rain kept pouring was challenging. I held my giant backpack behind me, my small pack in front of me, my ukulele draped over my shoulder, and my flashlight in one hand. I thought it might be safer to crawl, so I somehow managed to lower myself onto my hands and knees and took one step in this way. I quickly discovered that this was much more challenging while carrying all of my things. So I slowly and carefully stood back up and continued walking, one careful step after another. Each plank tested my limits, and the only thing that kept me going was focusing on advancing to the next piece of wood. I would occasionally zoom out to see the end of the bridge, which seemed so far away, and I would try to count how many steps were left. This seemed daunting and terrorizing. So, I zoomed back in to take the next step.

Finally, the end was near, and I felt my adrenaline begin to fade. I stepped on solid ground and could not believe I had crossed safely. I felt so powerful at that moment, unstoppable, impenetrable. I began to sing so loudly:

"Mírame bien, de más allá
Esta mujer tiene poder
La abuela luna ya me llamo
No estoy sola
El Gran Espíritu me adora
Take a look at me, further than the eye can see
This woman has power
The grandmother moon has already called me
I am not alone
The Great Spirit adores me"

I felt so blessed by my spirit guides and knew I was close to arriving at this community. After the bridge, I kept walking for a bit and saw no sign of anything that seemed like a community, so I continued walking for over an hour. Something seemed wrong since the entire journey was only supposed to take half an hour. So I became assured that I must have already passed it.

Arriving at a field with hundreds of cows, I suddenly found myself knee-deep in a pile of mud and cow poop. I didn't know whether to laugh or cry. So I did both. This seemed like a perfect moment to turn around. On my way back, I heard ferocious dogs barking. And while I did feel a bit threatened and intimidated by these dogs, I thought that perhaps where there were dogs, there were people. And people could offer me directions or a dry place to wait out the rain. As I approached the house where the dogs were, I tried announcing myself by shouting, *"Hola,"* but no one answered. I got close and peered in through the windows. It seemed that no one was home. I decided I would pitch my tent there and rest until morning.

The day had held enough adventure and mystery for me, and I surrendered to the powers of the rain making love to the dark night. I vowed to continue my search in the morning when the sun came out. I was getting ready to take out my tent when I found a little brick house and peeked inside to find that it was a chicken coop. I saw a small, flat, dry corner with hay that quickly became a tantalizing bed for the night. I took out my sleeping bag and tossed it on the hay pile next to the chickens. I removed my mud and cow poop-covered clothing and crawled into my sleeping bag. I must have been exhausted from the trek and the crashing adrenaline because I fell fast asleep. I had highly turbulent dreams all night, feeling the fear of arriving at some random person's house in the middle of the night in this small Colombian town I had never been to. But somehow, I slept through the night and awoke with the first rays of the sun.

I quickly gathered my things and peered out of the chicken coop to see if anyone was around. I noticed a woman milking cows down the hill, so I packed and ran toward her excitedly. She seemed confused about where I was coming from and how I had gotten there at six in the morning, so I explained my night's adventure to her. She was shocked! She told me that no one had crossed that bridge for hundreds of years, and since it was perilous, they had created a safer path off to the side. She told me that the house I slept in was home to an angry man who did not return home last night because he became too drunk and stayed in town. She also told me that she knew of the community I was trying to find and that I had passed it right after the second bridge. She said she was delivering milk in that direction, and we began walking together. We walked about one hour back in the opposite direction, and finally, I arrived. A sense of relief and gratitude washed over me.

Shortly after arriving, I met one of the few men who lived in this community of mostly women and children. He had a dark and secretive nature, and something about his energy felt familiar and even attractive to me. I hadn't yet begun my womb healing journey and was still resonating from a place of low self-worth. Unconsciously, I was still seeking toxic, manipulative encounters with men.

One night, this man invited me over to his cabin. Since I was the only volunteer and all of the families and children would typically wind down to bed early each evening, I would normally spend my evenings alone. So when he extended an invitation, I was open to sharing company with him.

When I came in, we chatted briefly, and he offered to massage me on his bed. I felt some creepiness but also lonely in this new community. The quality time I would share with the families during the day nourished me, but each family kept to themselves at night. Traveling alone in my early twenties, I craved intimate connections, loving affirmative touch, and socialization. So I surrendered to his massage, and shortly, I felt his energy become very aroused. Even though I didn't feel aroused or reciprocate any sexual attraction for this man, we spiraled into having penetrative sex.

This was by no means an assault because I consented to it. But my yes was passive, and I felt numb throughout the experience. I felt so detached from my body that I witnessed my lifeless self lying there as I looked over from above. I did not want him to penetrate me, but he did. And when he finished, everything was finished. I had this sense that he was somehow feeling lighter as if he had relieved himself of a heavy burden and had given it all to me. I was left with a feeling of disgust and emptiness. I didn't have to express my desire to leave his home as quickly as possible because he asked me to go immediately after finishing. He had gotten what he wanted and was ready to send me off.

As I lay alone in my tent that night, I vowed never to open myself sexually to this man again. I knew we would still have to live together in the community and perhaps remain friends or respectful neighbors, but the icky feeling I had in my womb affirmed that it was not safe or pleasurable for me to engage in sex with him. When we saw each other the next day, I instantly felt him go from 0 to 100 mph on the arousal dial. He grabbed my body and started squeezing my breasts and butt. It took me a little while to process what was happening, but eventually, I switched out of my paralysis and pushed him off me. He seemed alarmed that I was not excited to receive this sexual energy from him. He assumed that just because I had lent my body to him last night, I was somehow his property, readily available to be turned on whenever he wanted sex. I told him I did not want him to be sexual and needed him to respect my body and boundaries.

He responded dismissively, making it clear how little he cared about my boundaries and how disappointed he felt that he couldn't just have me sexually whenever he wanted. His response awoke a deep feeling of guilt that I somehow owed him my body. I feared he would lose interest in me altogether if I were unwilling to engage with him sexually. So why did I need to continue investing energy into this relationship if I felt unsafe, unworthy, and manipulated? I wish I could have seen clearly at the time that this man had a lot of shadows he was working through, and it was best to keep him at a distance while I worked through my shadows. But the unhealed sex trauma within my womb kept drawing me near him like a magnet.

I would still go to his house, making an excuse that the company was nice. But everything about it was secretive and clouded in shame. He always ensured that I would come over after dark so no one would see or know we were spending intimate time together. He made me promise not to tell anyone in the community what was happening between us. Whenever I came over, he would act aloof and indifferent, like he could care less if I came into his home. But I could sense his excitement on the inside, his eagerness to play with how much he could manipulate me. Yet he would never express his joy to see me externally. Instead, he would shroud this excitement in a protective mechanism of dismissal.

One night, I came over to his home, and he drew himself near me and began brushing my arm. I felt okay with that kind of touch, but then I felt him press his hard boner up against me. Instead of leaving, I tried to explain to someone who had already demonstrated that he did not understand a thing or two about consent that I was okay with arm scratches but not with the genitalia. This dance went on forever. He would calm down and pretend to be touching me without sexual expectations, but I would keep my guard up because eventually, he would reach for my breasts or try to kiss my neck, and I would feel the frustration growing within me. Yet I stayed, justifying that this was the kind of treatment I was worthy of. I can imagine how confusing it must have been for him as well. Because although I would say no with my words, my body would stay. So perhaps because I couldn't trust in my capacity to set clear boundaries, he too felt that he could easily violate my wavering no.

Eventually, after a handful of these events, I confided in a woman from the community and shared my feelings. I was not prepared for the response I received. She called on the community's women to join us in an emergency circle that night. There, I was asked to share with everyone what had occurred between this man and me, and as I spoke, I witnessed emotions of grief, anger, and compassion arise in these women. Then, all the stories poured out, with each one of the women in the circle sharing the ways this man had sexually terrorized them. They used the phrase "emotional terrorism" to express how they felt when, long after moving past traumatizing events with this man, they would feel his dark shadow continue to visit them and make them feel unsafe in their home. After many tears were shed, prayers were made, blessings for collective healing sent up to the creator, and we sang our hearts out to the beat of our medicine drums, the women felt it necessary to call in a community meeting where everyone could speak their truth into the light. This community was primarily women, but there were a few men and many children.

Everyone gathered a few days later to hold space to name how community members felt unsafe with this man's presence and to determine what action steps could be taken to create safety. As the circle began, I watched the children so the grownups could talk without needing the young ones to witness this entangled process. I am an educator with a talent for sinking into the present moment with children and giving them my undivided attention during our play and learning. However, this day, I couldn't focus on the children. Instead, I felt the tension of this circle emanating far beyond its container of bodies, and my stomach churned as I wondered what was occurring. It seemed to go on for hours until I eventually perceived that the circle had been completed because this man came walking straight toward me. He walked with conviction and asked me to step aside from the children so he could speak to me.

There was a blazing fire of rage inside his beady black eyes. His energy was threatening, precisely what he was hoping to achieve. He asked me why I had spread lies about him to the community since he was now asked to leave the space. He denied any sexual exchange between us and said it was my fault that he would have nowhere to live. I felt attacked, manipulated, and shamed for sharing my lived experience. I didn't feel safe having this conversation alone, and I told him that if he wanted to talk with me, it would have to be in front of the whole community. I marched over to the women who were still gathered and told them that he had already come angrily toward me in an attempt to silence me. Instead of taking responsibility for his actions and asking for forgiveness, he projected his guilt onto me and tried to pin me as the scapegoat. The women ignited like a forest fire on a hot summer day and immediately called everyone to join the circle. I don't know who watched the children at that time.

I sat directly across from this man. As I shared with the community what had been occurring between us, he shook his head in denial to assure (mostly the men he perceived as his allies) that my lived experience was invalid. I felt that sharing my story in this circle and witnessing my experience be denied was even more traumatic than when he sexually touched my body without my consent.

My womb hardened at that moment, holding on to this feeling that it was unsafe to share my stories and that I would have been better off keeping my mouth shut. Ultimately, it seemed pointless to work toward a communal growth and healing model when one of the humans was not ready to show up and do the work. So the meeting closed, and we knew our work lay within our wombs. To heal our bodies as womb keepers and support each other along the way was all we could do. To pray that our journey toward our center would contribute to our liberation and, in turn, continuously spiral outward for the benefit of all beings.

The women of this community took full accountability for supporting me in my womb-healing journey through the process of beginning to bleed again. I remember in one woman's circle, I couldn't stop crying. I felt cracked open and exposed as if I were a fragile little victim. An elder woman approached me and firmly held onto my shoulders while looking me in the eyes. With determination and compassion, she said, "I know you hold a lot of sexual trauma in your womb. Some of it is your own, and some of it is generational. But all the pain and the suffering you have already endured is part of your life path to support the healing of other womb keepers (*las guardianas de la vida*)."

I chuckled and scoffed at helpless little me empowering others to move through sexual trauma. Yet, I also received a clear vision in that moment. I was holding women's circles in my beautiful Earth-based home in the mountains, supporting womb keepers of all ages to reconnect to their cycle. The woman could sense the process she had ignited within me through her comment. She affirmed, "I want you to believe what I say because I commune with angels, and they showed me a clear vision of your most radiant, beautiful self transforming these wounds and supporting others. This is part of why you have been called on to this Earth. You will discover how to transmute the painful trauma into fulfillment, pleasure, and connection."

While I noticed the ever-present fear and doubt, I remained open to nurturing this curious seed within me and witnessed myself blossom into this decision. Finally, I felt ready to invite deep healing and cleansing of the trauma stored in my womb space.

Shortly after, I had my IUD removed.

One early morning, before the sun began to rise, a dear sister accompanied me to Bogota, leaving our mountain refuge for a day in the big city. We made an appointment at a Colombian version of Planned Parenthood, and they removed this little hormonal piece of plastic from my sacred center. When I came out of the procedure, my sister was waiting for me with flowers, and we jumped for joy in the waiting room. No one else in the space could have understood how pivotal this moment was for me. She then led me to a store where I bought my first menstrual cup and reusable cloth pads. She asked if my flow was typically heavy or light so I could decide what size cup to purchase. But I couldn't even remember since my last bleed had been so many years ago. I felt I was beginning anew, immersing myself in what felt like my first period.

This invitation allowed me to dive into a beautiful reconnection with myself, my body's cyclical nature, and the healing power of connecting to my menstrual blood: each cycle, a deeper understanding of the wisdom stored within me. I began building a bridge of connection with other cyclical women. As the moons passed, I played with creating different cyclical calendars and observing the changes in my physical and emotional body throughout my cycle. As I bled, I used my cup and filled up a small glass jar with my moon blood throughout my bleeding days. At the end of my menstruation, I often performed a ritual where I offered my blood back to Mother Earth, intending to release, transform, and rebirth.

While connecting to my cyclical magic served as a tool for my liberation and healing, inevitably, my journey included supporting other womb keepers to walk this healing path as well. So I began writing *Moon Blood*, a product of many years of my exploration, redesigning cyclical calendars, incorporating new embodied wisdom, trial and error, taking space, and coming back with the spiraling of cycles.

There has never been a more urgent time on this Earth for all womb keepers to reclaim their magic and honor themselves. As you honor your body, you act in sacred respect and reciprocity with the body of Mother Earth. She begs you to remember, listen to her, walk, dance, sing, and pray alongside her. The Great Mother, the infinitely fertile womb of creation for all life, birthed all beings on this Earth. As a womb keeper, you, too, carry an infinite potential to create and transform life.

Cross-culturally, women used to bleed together and honor their menstruation as a sacred time to allow their bodies to connect deeply with the Great Spirit. Unfortunately, many of us have forgotten the potent power of this magic, and most bleeding bodies are not given the time and space to sink into slowness, prayer, and ritual during their bleed time. Taking this moment to pause and reset with each moon cycle is essential for your overall health and wellness. Ultimately, the more you can slow down and recharge during your bleeding days, the more you can fully blossom into your beautiful, abundant fertility during your ovulation days.

The Earth is calling for your blood. This is why many ancient practices included animal sacrifices to offer the internal waters that sustain life back to the Earth. Unfortunately, planet Earth is plagued by wars, crime, violence, and mindless bloodshed. I believe that if every womb keeper offered their blood back to Mother Earth each month, there would cease to be violent bloodshed of human lives.

Your menstrual blood is infinitely wise and powerful. The blood from your uterine lining contains information about your lineage, stored collective memories, high iron and nitrogen content, and even stem cells. Observing your blood and noticing its transformations throughout the cycles is a sacred radical ritual of reconnection to yourself and your ancestors. Imagine that when your grandmother was born, she already carried all of the eggs she could fertilize throughout her life within her womb. Eventually, one of those eggs became your mother, who birthed you. So everything that may have impacted your grandmother in her physical body, emotional trauma, habitual patterns, etc., is directly stored as cellular memory in your womb space. This is not to say that you are a victim of your past, but simply recognizing your past as a part of you is an extremely powerful component of your path toward self-discovery and liberation.

I want to support you in tuning into the wise messages your womb is whispering to you.

I want to support you in reclaiming your womb, a place that has collectively stored trauma, abuse, pain, sickness, wounds, violation, abortion, shame, toxic chemicals, and silencing, as a place of creation, fertility, intuition, magic, deeply embodied pleasure, remembering, wisdom, liberation, beauty, and reconnection.

One womb keeper waking up to their power is huge, and this healing has the potential to ripple infinitely outward and expand toward all beings. Queen Afua, in her book *Sacred Woman: A Guide to Healing The Feminine Mind, Body, Spirit*, says, "Know that wherever a woman is healing her womb, there is a household for the potential of healing and wellness. One household at a time, prayerfully, this healing will spread like a cleansing fire throughout the world's communities."

Prioritizing womb healing will support you in designing your life around the ebbs and flows of your cycle and work with her magic.

Through cycle tracking, you will become autonomous over your fertility and can use this wisdom for contraception or conception without needing hormonal birth control.

You will rise into your most empowered self and connect to other womb keepers, awakening to their inner wisdom and weaving this web together.

You will explore regulating your cycle and entering your body's natural rhythm.

You will explore how to live harmoniously with your body's natural cyclical rhythm.

You will experience (mostly) pain-free periods. In addition, you will learn how to use food and medicinal herbs to support each stage of your cycle and design a cyclical body movement plan aligned with your hormonal shifts.

As you heal your womb, you heal our Earth. The Great Mother, alongside infinite seen and unseen forces, calls you to return, remember, and reclaim your divinity. Are you ready and open to receiving this wisdom? She is singing deep within your sacred center, the same as Mother Earth's sacred center.

Are you listening?

Womb Magic

"This chain of womb unwellness cannot come to an end until you realize that you're the only one who can change the whole energy pattern... there is a light [in you] that refuses to be turned down or off, no matter how the whole family has been functioning for hundreds of years... you are one of the medicine woman the whole planet has been waiting for – waiting for you to remember, to bring forth Earth wisdom once more" ~ Queen Afua

Before diving deeper into womb wellness and the magic stored within these pages, now would be a great moment to pause and check in with your womb.

❭ Do you feel her pulsating inside of you?

❭ Does she feel tense?

❭ Is she open and trusting?

❭ What stories is she holding on to?

When these women first asked me to meditate with my womb in Colombia, I couldn't feel anything. I had this sensation of searching for a needle in a haystack while being sucked through an infinitely vast black hole. How could I focus on the sensations of my womb when this had been a place of numbness for so long? These women encouraged me to be patient and loving with myself, reminding me that simply investing the effort to sense my womb within my body was already strengthening the connections that had laid dormant for so long.

One night, as I lay there trying to tune into my womb, I felt tight, like she was clinging to something for dear life. I wondered what would happen if I tried to let go. So, just as if I were trying to release tension with any muscle in my body,

I released the tension in my womb and felt an orgasmic flood of spaciousness flow through me. I was elated. It was as if I had a micro orgasm within. After endless hours of meditating with my womb and feeling nothing, I finally felt her respond to my presence. I knew this journey would be slow, but I felt hopeful and curious to continue exploring what else I could discover within my body.

Here are some questions you can weave into your meditation or sit with as journal prompts. Take this time to authentically listen to your womb without expecting how she may respond. Sending you blessings as you begin this journey!

- Ask your womb why you may have never conversed with her before.

- How have you silenced your womb?

- What do you need to feel supported to heal your womb?

- What is your current relationship to your menstrual cycle?

- Do you have a personal practice you honor during your bleed days?

- How did you feel about your first menstruation?

- How did you feel about your first sexual intercourse?

- How do you feel about sex now?

- Do you currently have the capacity to listen to and trust your intuitive wisdom?

- Are there any stories of trauma (either from your lifetime, your mother, or grandmother) stored within your womb that you are curious about exploring?

- Do you have a personal pleasure practice?

☽ What is your relationship to your expression of gender?

☽ What is your relationship to your sexual orientation?

☽ In what ways do you express your creativity?

☽ Do you have a Spirit guide? In what ways does this Spirit communicate with you?

☽ Do you have an important dream or vision waiting to manifest?

☽ What does freedom feel like within your body?

☽ In what ways would you like to be supported during your moon phases, ranging from menstruation to ovulation?

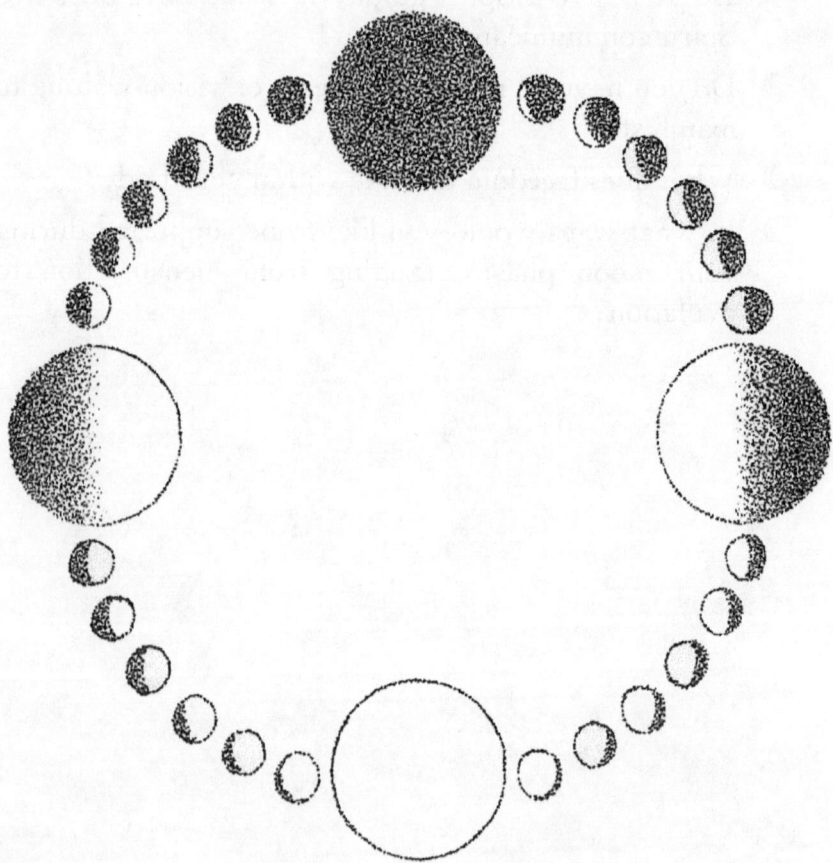

Menstruation and the Moon

"The moon is Earth's oldest temple holding the poetry of countless prayers since the dawn of time... a bell whose ringing brings you into the field of the Mother where body and soul can quietly drink."~ Dana Gerhardt, author of Mooncircles.

The moon is in a constant state of transformation. It rebirths itself approximately every 28-29 days as it enters a new moon cycle. The moon is eternally dancing with all forms of water and strongly affects the ebb and flow of the tides. Millions of years ago, when the moon was much closer to the Earth, our planet was covered in a giant ocean of crashing waves. As the moon gradually drifted farther from Earth, the seas calmed, land formed, and the moon took its distant home in the sky. With their divine placement in space, the moon and the Earth continue their ever-evolving relationship. As the cycles of the moon change, everything on Earth moves according to its rhythm. Since the moon affects water, and much of life on Earth is made up of water, the moon's phases affect us internally. We humans are 70% water! As the moon grows into its whole state, energy is heightened and can lead to a wild animalistic awakening (hence the term lunatic, coming from the Latin word for moon—*luna*).

While the moon's cycles affect all living beings on Earth, a long-standing ancestral pact exists between cyclical beings who bleed monthly and the moon's cycles. Menstruation is a powerful portal to connect to new moon energy in a bleeding person's body. With every new moon, your body is given the opportunity to let go and rebirth from your sacred womb space. Once you deconstruct shame, disgust, and the lack of connection you may have felt about your menstruation, you can begin interacting with your moon blood from a place

5

of compassion and curiosity, tapping into your truest magic. Your menstrual blood is a crucial indicator of your overall health and can reveal wisdom about what is happening in your inner world.

There are many ancient cultural traditions in which women were excluded from certain rituals when they were with their moon because the menstruation ritual is already so powerful that it must be given the time and space to reveal itself. For example, many South American shamans will not allow a woman with her moon to join ceremony because her energy is so strong at this time that it may take him out of his center. Additionally, in Jewish traditions, women were excluded from cooking, child-rearing, and typical household duties because they were supposedly "impure" in those days. So women would create red tents to join and spend their bleeding days together, nurturing each other, elevating their collective prayers, resting, and connecting to their truest wisdom. They could retreat in these tents and let their bodies naturally cleanse themselves. Other women would serve the bleeding bodies by massaging them, preparing meals and drinks, sharing stories, and holding ceremony. In Native American traditions, women would vision these days since they were most open to connecting to spirit. Then, the tribe would receive these women's visions as guidance for the community. In many nomadic cultures, menstruating women would gather together and envision where to lead their tribe.

I like to believe that women's magic was incomprehensible to men in those days, so in their intimidation of these women's infinite power, they would give her the space to honor her moon time. Therefore, it is not that bleeding bodies are incapable of joining in other rituals during this time; instead, it is an opportunity for bleeding bodies to be with themselves in their raw and sacred state, which is a ritual in and of itself.

Overview of the Menstrual Cycle

My exploration of the synchronous cycles of the moon and menstruation centers heavily on the energetics of each phase (which we will dive deeper into later). Therefore, while I do not intend to explore the specific intricacies of hormonal changes throughout the cycle, I will share a brief overview of some of the changes occurring in a menstruating body over the course of one complete cycle.

The cycle begins on the first day of bleeding, typically lasting 3-5 days (although all bodies are unique). During menstruation, estrogen and progesterone are at an all-time low, and your body releases many nutrients and minerals while breaking down your uterine lining. This is a time to cleanse, hydrate, rest, and restore.

Once bleeding has ceased, you move into the follicular phase, which typically lasts 4-7 days. In this phase, estrogen begins to rise to support the building of the endometrium, stimulate the production of fertile cervical fluid, and increase libido. While all bodies are different, typically after menstruation, there will be a few days of no cervical fluid production, referred to as dry days. As estrogen rises, there may start to be a change in cervical fluid production from some baseline fluid (nothing, dry, crumbly, creamy, gluey) to fertile cervical fluid (sticky, milky, boogery, slick, transparent).

In this preovulatory follicular phase, your basal body temperature remains low. You can explore your basal body temperature by keeping a thermometer by your bed (one that reads for at least 30 seconds) and taking your temperature orally every morning (ideally at the same time each day, between 5-8 a.m.). You will start to note your typical low temperatures and high temperatures throughout your cycle. Your temperature should remain on the low side throughout the ovulatory phase, which typically lasts 3-5 days (although the actual release of the egg in the ovulation process typically only lasts 24 hours).

Once you notice that your temperature has risen due to the rise in progesterone, you can confirm that ovulation has already occurred. Although you can energetically feel that you are ovulating by noticing your mood, your sexual desire, your cervical fluids, and your cervix position, you can only confirm that you have ovulated by seeing a high temperature the following day. And if you are hoping to have sex not for conception, it is recommended that you wait for four consecutive days of a higher temperature before having safe penetrative sex. This phase is known as the luteal phase.

Your luteal phase typically lasts 12-14 days, including the post-ovulatory and premenstrual phases. With increased progesterone levels, your cervical fluid will begin to dry, and your body will prepare to menstruate again. Your temperature will remain high this second half of your cycle and will only drop back down on the day of or before your next menstruation. You will know that your body will bleed again and that all reproductive hormones are at an all-time low because you may begin to feel heavy and have low energy. Taking your temperature is a helpful tool to confirm you have ovulated and let you know that your moon is coming.

Seed Cycling

A suggested practice to regulate your hormones (specifically the ebbs and flows of estrogen and progesterone) and truly connect to your food as medicine is seed cycling. Seed cycling is a simple yet potent practice of incorporating raw seeds into your diet according to the phase of your cycle. While the menstrual cycle contains four phases, the seed cycles can be divided into two phases.

In seed cycling, the first phase begins at menstruation and continues until ovulation. In this phase, estrogen rises within the body, so flax and pumpkin seeds are ideal to incorporate into your diet to balance estrogen levels. Flaxseeds contain phytoestrogens, which produce an estrogen-like effect on the body. They also contain lignans, which absorb excess estrogen. Pumpkin seeds are high in zinc, an essential mineral in forming the corpus luteum. The corpus luteum thickens the uterus lining for potential implantation and progesterone production.

The second phase begins at ovulation and continues through the premenstrual phase until menstruation. In this phase, progesterone rises, so sunflower and sesame seeds are ideal to bring balance to the body. Sunflower seeds are high in selenium, which supports the liver to detox any extra estrogen. Sesame seeds are also high in lignans, which balance estrogen and progesterone levels. Both sunflower and sesame seeds contain high levels of omega-6, an essential fatty acid for hormone production and follicle function.

When practicing seed cycling, consuming the seeds raw, untoasted is important. I prefer to activate the seeds in a glass of water overnight and consume them in the morning either on their own, blended into a smoothie, or mixed into oats. For quantities, I suggest listening to your body and making accommodations for your needs. A rough guide can be one heaping spoonful of each daily, leading to two spoonfuls of raw, preferably soaked, seeds daily. Flax and pumpkin in the first phase. Sunflower and sesame in the second phase. If you cannot access all four seeds, I still believe even incorporating one of these seeds into your diet benefits hormone regulation. If you want to try the complete seed cycle, I recommend trying 2-3 menstrual cycles of seed cycling to witness its effect on your body. Some changes occur immediately; others, like perhaps hormone imbalances, are deeply rooted and require some patience. Trust in the process and do your best to remain diligent. And if you forget a day or two, this is a wonderful opportunity to practice self-compassion and forgiveness and to dive right back in.

Shed, Release, Transform

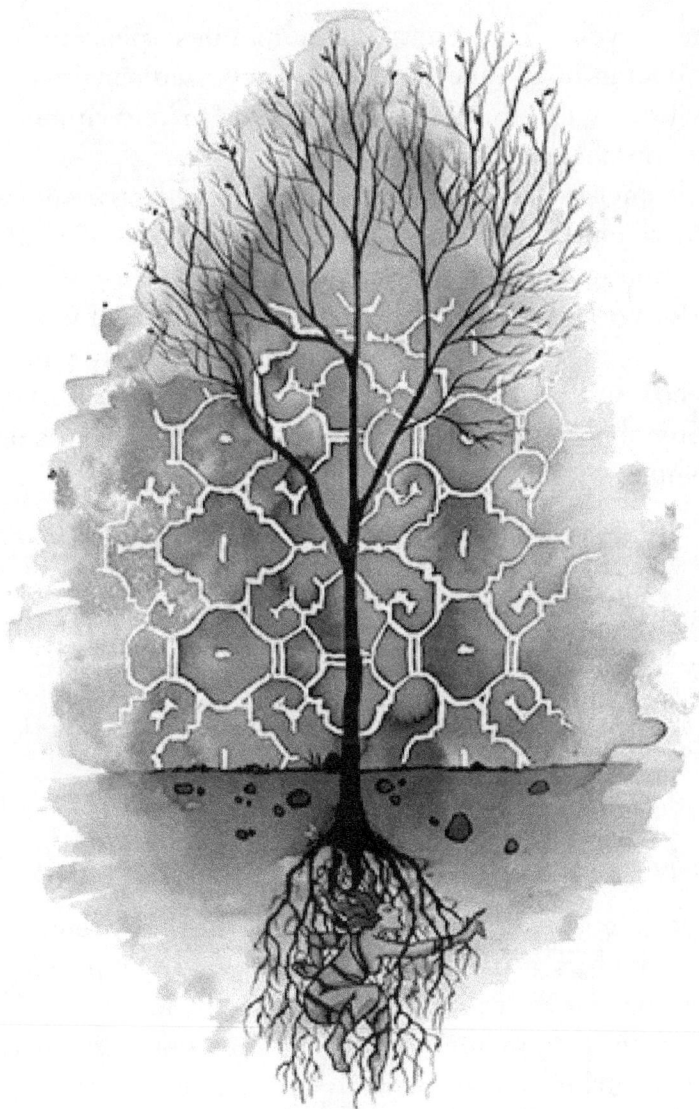

Moon's Energy

As the moon winds down into darkness, approximately from days 21-28 of the moon cycle, this waning stage is a powerful time to release, transform, and create space for the new cycle. This energy can manifest peacefully, like experiencing heightened intuition, increased sensitivity, and wise witchy wisdom. This is a great time to hold rituals, build altars, and channel divine messages.

This energy can also manifest in wildly destructive ways, like the raging waters of a tsunami, the eruption of a volcano, the trembling of an earthquake, and the whirling winds of a tornado. We possess all of the powers of Mother Earth within our bodies, and just as we are capable of lovingly tending to our seeds and nurturing them to life, we are also capable of passionately lighting a fire to all that no longer serves us and nourishing the soil for the future seeds to come.

Moon Phase: Waning Moon

The Waning Moon is the last quarter of this cycle, allowing us to close any projects we began in this moon cycle and prepare for the upcoming dark New Moon.

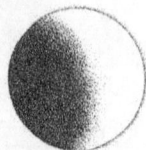

Menstrual Cycle Phase: Premenstrual

This menstrual phase connects to the premenstrual phase, which is a part of the luteal phase. Your body has been preparing your uterine lining with the loving conditions required to sustain life. Assuming that your egg was not fertilized during ovulation, your body is preparing to break down the uterine lining and release all of this life-force energy back to the Earth.

There is so much magic, grief, and transformation within you at this time of the cycle. Without acknowledging this intense power, your body may react in wildly unpredictable ways. The premenstrual phase has notoriously been referred to as an irritable and bitchy phase because if you do not hold space for the internal chaos to flow through your creative being, you may begin to feel anxious and project this outwardly. Perhaps as you start to track your cycle, simply creating space to observe, write down the sensations, and release judgments on the emotions that arise for you in this time may give you the confidence to best support and meet your premenstrual needs.

Since this is a highly intuitive time in which you are open to receiving messages from your body, you may feel called to travel inward and protect your energy from external influences. This is your time to discover what you desire to release and set that clear intention to prepare for your upcoming menstruation. Allow this time to be an invitation to sit with all of you (yes, your shadow self, too) and compassionately observe any feelings that may arise. Invite your wounds into your meditations, your prayers, your body movement, your verbal expression, your writing practice, and into your creative processes. Remember that there is nothing inside or outside of you to feel shame about. After all, we do not shame the moon for waning. We witness its ebb and flow and learn to work with her magic.

In my premenstrual experience, I often feel irritable, exhausted, anxious, sad, sensitive, creative, increased libido, intuitive, slow, sensual, and introverted. (At times, just one of these sensations or a wild potion of them all!) However, I have found that I can often tap into wildly powerful creative magic in this phase by creating a compassionate container to witness and release whatever needs to flow through me.

Cervical Dance

During this premenstrual phase, you may note cervical fluids ranging from creamy, sticky, lotiony, crumbly, wet, or even dry. While cervical fluids constantly change throughout your cycle, the position and texture of the cervix is also shifting. However, all bodies are different, so by tracking your cycle, you will notice patterns and changes in your cervical fluid throughout your cycle. Whether you stick a clean finger up your vagina a few times a day or observe your underwear or toilet paper when wiping, you will open an intimate conversation with your womb about the processes occurring within.

While cervical fluids constantly change throughout your cycle, their position and texture are also constantly shifting. You are no longer fertile in this premenstrual phase, so your cervix will take on a low, firm, closed position.

Season: Fall

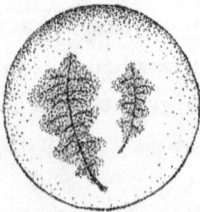

The corresponding season is Fall when the warm summer nights turn to chilly evenings, and all leaves begin their dance down toward Mother Earth. This is your body's time to transition from the height of summer extroversion to the dark depths of winter introspection.

Element: Earth

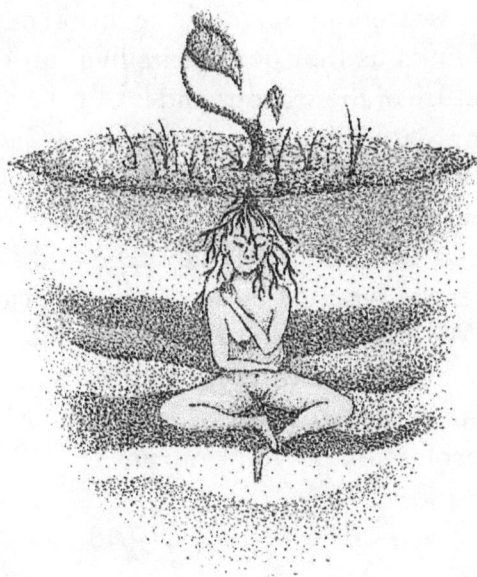

The corresponding element is Earth. This is your time to find grounding and sink into your roots. As trees shed their leaves, the only thing that will sustain them through the cold winter is relying on the support of their roots firmly drawing in nourishment from Mother Earth.

This is a potent time to examine how to cultivate more groundedness within your body temple and throughout your life.

Weave stones and roots into your meditations, get your hands in the soil, play with clay, and meditate with crystals. Connect with the divine element of Earth that makes up all life, including your womb, plants, and animals. We are all made up of the same celestial stardust.

Direction: West

Each one of these phases corresponds to one of the four directions. In the Native American medicine wheel, also known as the sacred hoop, a circle broken up into four quadrants reminds us that our spirits live forever, similar to the circular nature of the seasons and life cycles. The direction we are opening with this phase is the West Gate, associated with black. This direction begins our death process so that we can later be reborn. This is a powerful time to examine the parts of yourself that bring self-sabotage and hold space for deep, old ancestral wounds you wish to release. The power animal of the West is the Jaguar, who embodies fearlessness, honors her instinctive, intuitive nature, and knows what must die for other life to carry on. The Jaguar is a symbol of courage and protection on your journey.

Astrological Signs

The moon moves through a new astrological sign within this grand mandala every 2-3 days. Since the moon relates to the Earth in 28-day cycles, there will typically be a new moon in a specific astrological sign on day one and a full moon in its complementary opposing astrological sign on day 14. Since there are 12 signs that the moon will move through in each 28-day moon cycle, the moon is moving through a new sign approximately every 2-3 days.

We tend to note the sign that the full moon and new moon occur since these energies are the most heightened and can be felt with more clarity. Yet, the astrological sign that the moon is in daily also reveals how the moon constantly affects your emotions throughout your cycle. (Here is a little tip: I use an incredible app called Astrovizor, which I tune into daily, and I can see at any given moment where the moon is, as well as track the movement of many other celestial bodies.)

I draw wisdom from Western Astrology, and for this mandala, I invite you to observe the moon's movement and note how it affects your internal emotional, feminine, receptive state. If observing the astrological signs is an entirely new concept for you, I encourage you to take it slow and allow yourself to notice any patterns without seeking any specific outcomes. On the other hand, if you are an astrological expert, perhaps you may note how the movement of other celestial bodies, their aspects, or their house placement interact with your cyclical flow. When I began to make note of the changing signs, I focused on the element of the sign and observed how the energetics of that element shaped the expression of my emotional state on that given day.

Since there are 12 astrological signs and four elements, there are three signs in each element:

☽ Fire Signs: Aries, Leo, Sagittarius

☽ Earth Signs: Taurus, Virgo, Capricorn

☽ Air Signs: Gemini, Libra, Aquarius

☽ Water Signs: Cancer, Scorpio, Pisces

Additionally, each sign contains a particular cardinal, fixed, or mutable quality. Since there are 12 astrological signs and three qualities, each quality has four signs:

☽ Cardinal Signs: Aries, Taurus, Gemini, Cancer

☽ Fixed Signs: Leo, Virgo, Libra, Scorpio

☽ Mutable Signs: Sagittarius, Capricorn, Aquarius, Pisces

Cardinal signs initiate and begin a cycle, so when the moon is in a cardinal sign, this energy may support you in creating a new beginning in an aspect of your internal or external world.

Fixed signs sustain and nourish, so when the moon is in a fixed sign, this may support you in finding focus and endurance in following through with a project, relationship, or vision and preparing for the harvest.

Finally, mutable signs carry the energy of completion and transition, so when the moon is in a mutable sign, you may find an opportunity to reflect, look ahead, and sink into a feeling of flexibility and adaptability.

To flow with the four main components of this book, I have divided the twelve astrological signs into four sections in correspondence with their element. In this phase, I will give a brief overview of the Earth signs.

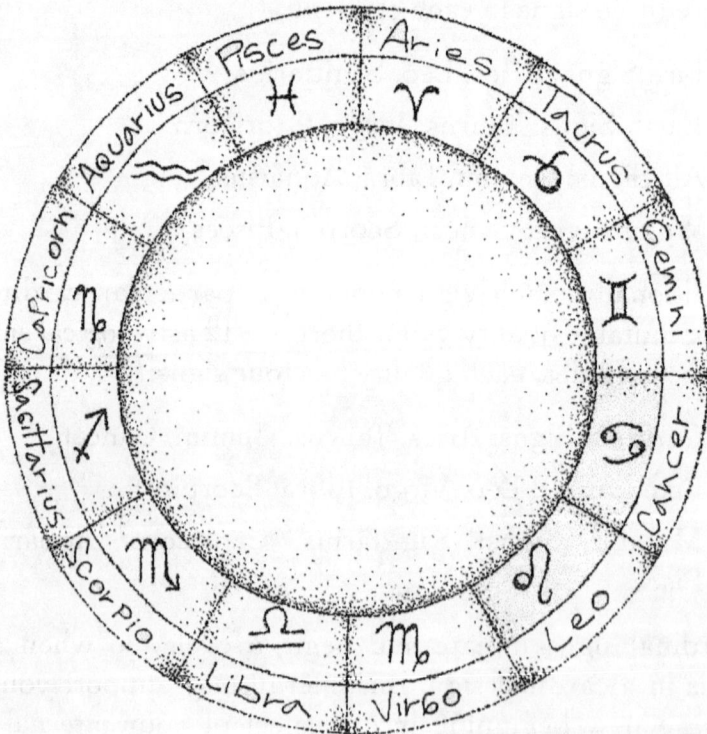

Earth Signs

Taurus: The second Zodiac sign, Taurus, is a cardinal Earth sign ruled by Venus, which tends to invite a sensual experience in this Earthly material world. The energy of Taurus makes space to enjoy physical comforts, engage all of the senses, and seek pleasure connected to your most authentic desires. Root into this sign's determined and focused strengths without becoming stubborn or seeking control. Remember to invite in balance and avoid overindulgence.

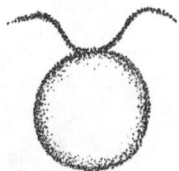

Virgo: The sixth Zodiac sign, Virgo is the second Earth sign, a fixed sign ruled by Mercury. This is a beautiful portal to gain mental clarity, bring physical order to your space, and dive into academic learning. Notice Virgo's tendency to be overly critical and invite in Virgo's qualities of hard work, dedication, organized categorization, and orientation toward details. Virgos are recognized as pure healers, so take this time to connect to your own medicine and bring healing and harmony to yourself and others.

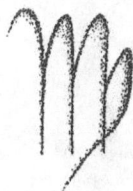

Capricorn: Capricorn is the tenth sign of the Zodiac, the third and final Earth sign, and a mutable sign ruled by Saturn. Capricorn energy is structured, loyal, responsible, and ambitious, representing the father's energy. This is a great time to focus on projects that require hard work and determination. However, this energy may sometimes move toward over-rigidity or austerity, so practice patience and balance while maintaining your independence.

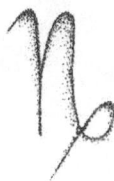

Female Archetype: Kali & Witch

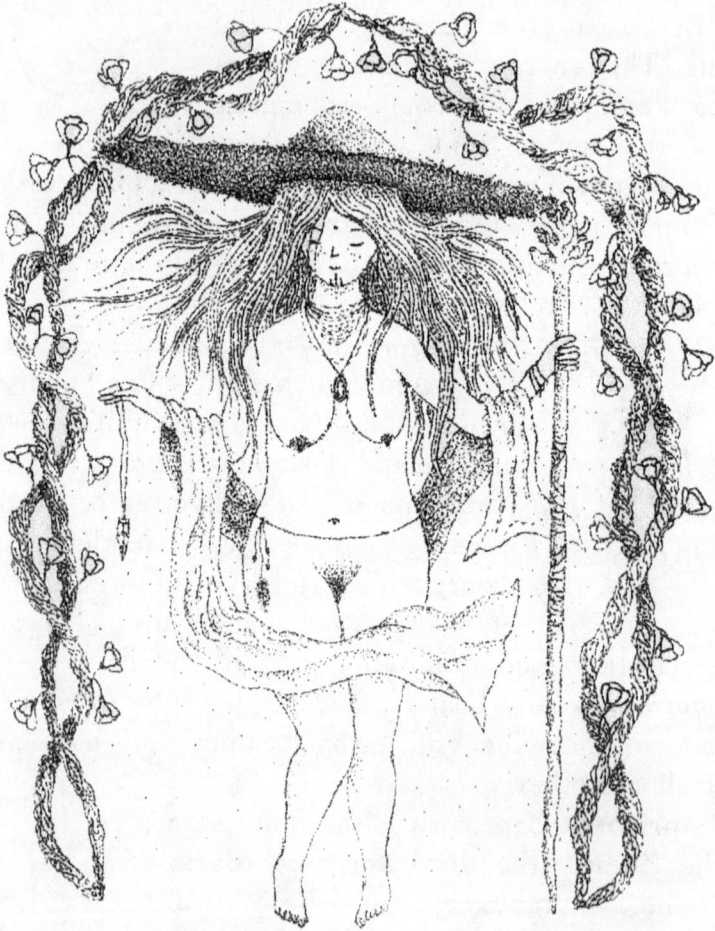

While several interpretations of the female archetypes are connected to each phase, I will offer the archetypes that most resonate with my cyclical journey.

In this premenstrual, waning moon phase, it is helpful to imagine embodying the archetype of Kali, the Indian Goddess of death, destruction, and creation. She has been depicted as a slayer of demons, unleashing her fully wild, savage, animalistic instincts to tap into the pleasure of destruction and transformation. This is the time to give yourself permission to be your wildest self. Find healthy ways to channel your destruction energy into creation energy. Perhaps you feel called to light candles in your dark room and dance naked. Maybe you feel called to run naked through the forest. Perhaps you feel like writing a wild erotic story late into the night. Find a practice that supports your need to express and release, withholding judgment about what emerges throughout the process. If an intuitive spark flows through you, listen to the message!

Clarissa Pinkola Estes, author of *Women Who Run With the Wolves*, describes this so poetically as she writes, "A woman may crave to be near water, or belly down, her face in the Earth, smelling the wild smell. She might have to drive into the wind. She may have to plant something, pull things out of or put them into the ground. She may have to knead and bake, rapped in dough up to her elbows. She may have to trek into the hills, leaping from rock to rock and trying out her voice against the mountain. She may need hours of starry nights where the stars are like face powder split on a black marble floor. She may feel she will die if she doesn't dance naked in a thunderstorm, sit in perfect silence, and return home ink-stained, paint-stained, tear-stained, moon-stained."

This is also the time to honor your inner witch, *bruja*. By using the word witch, you reclaim the magic you carry within, releasing any shame or fear attached to that word. Witch comes from the word "wit," meaning wise, and instead of being a denigrating word, it was used initially to name young and old female healers. When I attended protests in Chile, the women would scream on the streets, "*somos las nietas de las brujas que no pudiste quemar*... we are the granddaughters of the witches you could not burn." I invite you to fully embody your inner witch in whatever way feels authentic. Hold rituals, elevate your prayers, create magic potions, make spells for healing, and howl at the moon. Trust in your truth and honor your magic.

"Your womb is a treasure chest waiting to be explored. So open it up. See what intuitive gems of wisdom await you as you discover yourself by bringing what's inside... out! Your womb desires to speak through you. Your womb will tell you what she needs. Your womb will tell you where she's going and where she's been. Your womb will tell you how she wants to heal." Queen Afua

Suggested Foods

This is an important moment of your cycle to nourish yourself with foods rich in protein, omega-3, complex carbs, and fiber. Vitamin D (soaking up the sun's rays or consuming fish) balances mood swings, and vitamin B-6 (found in sunflower seeds, lentils, and brown rice) supports overall hormonal balance by helping the body produce serotonin. You may notice that you indulge in cravings and eat more in the premenstrual state as if your body knows that the winter hibernation is coming and, like a wise mama bear, is storing up for the winter.

Suggested Movement Plan

Before bleeding, your body creates more cortisol and progesterone in this phase. With increased levels of these hormones, it is not supportive to do high-intensity muscle-building exercises since you may burn through your muscle mass. On the other hand, this is the phase in which your body burns the most calories, so it is a great moment to incorporate long-endurance cardio. Find an activity you love most, like going on a hike, a run, a bike ride, or a swim, or put on your favorite playlist and dance around and get sweaty. Allow the serotonin and dopamine that your body produces through exercise wash over you like a calming rain to your premenstrual fires. As you get closer to your bleed and your body begins to feel heavy, slow, or sluggish, give yourself permission to slow down and prepare for the winter rest.

Suggested Herbal Support

For further support in releasing, detoxing, and purifying the body, try incorporating Dandelion (roots and greens) or Stinging Nettle. Nettle is rich in minerals, high in iron, and helps detox the kidney, making it a beautiful herbal accompaniment for the whole cycle. These herbs purify the blood and detoxify the liver. Detoxifying your blood in the premenstrual phase is crucial for a more easeful, pain-free menstruation.

If you want to add more fuel to this fiery moment of release, try incorporating some Ginger, Turmeric, and Cinnamon medicine. The ginger will revitalize and energize the womb with her heat. The turmeric will serve as an anti-inflammatory, easing any premenstrual bloating. The cinnamon will add a bit of sweetness, warmth, and balance. If you want something to reduce this phase's intensity, try incorporating some Lemon Balm, Calendula, Chamomile, or St. John's Wort for a calming, soothing, nervine medicine. These suggested herbs can be used as an oil, tincture, tea, or sprinkled into herbal baths.

Cyclical Gardening

Since the moon affects all life on Earth, it is supportive to tend to your gardens in sacred harmony with the moon's rhythms. Imagine the water flow constantly cycling up and down each plant through every moon cycle. During the waning moon, the waters are making their way down the stem or trunk of the plant so that the energy can arrive at the roots for the new moon. So, if you are trying to pull weeds out of your garden, they will likely not grow back if you can remove them in this phase. It is also an excellent time to harvest wood that you may use for building since the trunk is full of power. This is an ideal moment to transplant anything since the plant will continue to send power down to its roots as it situates itself in its new home.

The waning moon is also the best time to propagate plants. If you are new to propagation, imagine this. It's like going up to a human, chopping off their arm, and watching how this arm begins to grow feet, a head, and legs. From one limb, it becomes an entirely new human. In the context of humans, it sounds like a crazy science fiction movie, but for plants, it is truly a miraculous way of reproducing themselves. Propagation works great for creating an abundance of herbs in your garden. You can take a pair of scissors and chop some of the plant's stems, place them in a cup of water, and watch these stems grow new roots! As the moon gets closer and closer to a dark new moon, in the day or two before, it is best to let your garden rest. Just as your body rests in the upcoming menstruation, the Earth rests too in the days leading up to the new moon.

Writing Reflections

❱ In what ways can you unapologetically destroy, release, and transform something in your life right now?

❱ What do you need to feel safe to embody the pleasure of the transformation process fully?

❱ How can you honor your body's needs in this phase by meeting these needs on your own or asking for the support you desire?

❱ Where is there space right now to nourish fertile soil for the upcoming cycle?

❱ Where is there a resistance to release, and what do you need to nurture that resistance with loving compassion?

❱ Where is the root of your shadowy fears coming from so that you may pull it out and no longer own it?

❱ What supports you to feel grounded and rooted?

❱ What are safe, creative ways you can channel your wild Kali destructive energy?

Guided Fear Burning & Shaking Ritual

A helpful way to support your body to shed, release, and transform in this premenstrual phase is to work with the element of fire. Yes, while the corresponding element of this phase is the Earth element, we can always lean into the medicine of any of the four elements in any of the four phases.

First, create a sacred fire and hold space for this ritual alone or with friends. When your fire has been fully stoked, reflect with paper and pen on the following question.

❱ What fears, in this present moment, are limiting you from growing and evolving?

Feel free to write from your ego, the one who feels like the victim, the one who likes to suffer, the one who feels that the weight of the world rests on your shoulders.

Read through what you have written out loud, and now, you can reexamine those fears and write from your highest self, the wise one who can see the whole picture, the one who trusts in the divine plan, the one who offers guidance and comfort. Once all your fears, worries, and doubts have been put on paper, you acknowledge them, recognize their validity, and rewrite your story. Perhaps you visit a fear and rephrase it by saying, "Even though I am afraid of... I know that..." or "Even though I am worried about... my highest self trusts that..." or "Even though I criticize myself for... my wisest self knows that...."

In this exercise, you are allowing yourself to recognize your fears, validate and hold space for them, and withhold any judgment. You allow your fears to be seen by giving them a voice and releasing them onto your paper. And you can rewrite your story. Since your words, thoughts, and perceptions shape your reality, you can tune into the wisdom within you for guidance. Often, you may look for answers externally when your inner wisdom holds so much richness. Your intuition is powerful in this premenstrual phase, so it is vital to listen to yourself.

Once you have written your victim story, and then you have rewritten your story from your highest self, you can prepare to practice detachment and offer this paper to the fire. You may want to ask the element of fire to accompany your transformation process and to help you shed all that you no longer need. Once you have freed yourself from your fears, worries, burdens, and insecurities, it is time to bring this awareness fully into your body through movement.

Find a comfortable standing position near the fire and begin by feeling your feet rooted into the ground. Notice the sensations in your body without judging them. Scan yourself from head to toe, checking in with sensations on your skin, muscles, and bones. Once you have fully scanned your body, allow a wave of relaxation to wash over you, completely releasing any stored tension. Release your jaw. Soften your knees. Release tension in your sexual organs. And take in plenty of air. You can begin to incorporate a soft bounce of the knees and tune in to the natural rhythm of your body and breath to determine how slow, fast, small, or large your movement would be.

Bouncing your knees can invite bouncing and shaking to other parts of your body, like your feet, hands, shoulders, pelvis, and neck. Allow any stuck and pent-up energy to move through you freely. Allow your body to release any sounds that would like to emerge. Your voice is an expression of your body and a powerful tool to move energy within. If you start to feel tired, allow this bounce to energize you, knowing that you can draw energy up from the Earth and that you are constantly exchanging energy with the grandfather fire. Allow this movement to be your medicine. Don't hold anything back. Allow all stagnant energy to flow freely. Connect to the heat flowing within you. Once you feel complete, gradually slow your bouncing and clean your body with your hands, wiping and brushing off anything left behind by throwing it into the fire.

Notice what has shifted within your body.

⟩ How does your body feel now compared to when you scanned your body before shaking?

⟩ How does your body feel now compared to when you were beginning to light your fire?

Register any sensations, discoveries, and stories that emerge from your cellular memory. You can close this ritual by offering sage, cedar, lavender, palo santo, or copal (any incense that feels resonant to you) to the fire. Feel free to sing to the fire, keep writing, sit in stillness, or have a dance party. Listen to your body and trust your intuition.

Stories

In each section, I have included personal stories from my journey that reflect moments in my life in which I embodied each particular phase. I feel that it is incredibly vulnerable to tell my narrative in this way, and it also anchors the wisdom I share about the explorations I have made throughout my moon cycles. I know that I am not a professional "menstruologist," but I am a human who has been tracking my cycles and observing my ebbs and flows for many years. I am a human who has experienced sexual assault and is constantly spiraling toward healing my womb. I am a human who has lived in many different parts of the world, and I carry a unique cross-cultural richness. I am a human who has been supported by countless angels, guiding my way back home.

Reclaiming our narratives is a huge step toward decolonizing knowledge. Our knowledge does not come solely from academic or scientific studies. Our life experience is the juicy, messy, raw goodness that feeds our soul and gives meaning to this wisdom put into an embodied practice.

Throughout these reflections, I revisit parts of myself clouded in shame, guilt, rejection, grief, and self-doubt. I also revisit parts of myself that have felt complete empowerment, self-trust, deep embodied pleasure, transformations, rebirths, and striking clarity. Writing these stories has been profoundly healing. My intention in sharing them is that by reading some of my cyclical waves, you may feel a sense of inspiration, compassion, and self-empowerment. May you also gain the courage to share your story.

Let Go of Your Shit

Letting go is hard for me.

When I was sixteen, I began having horrible digestive issues. I would cycle through days of painful constipation and then release explosive diarrhea. Typically, in my family, when something was wrong with our health, we would see a Western medical doctor. Everyone in my family trusted their health to the pharmaceutical companies. My grandparents even owned a pharmacy in Mexico. My mom and I began to visit endless endocrinologists for months, during which I got numerous endoscopies and colonoscopies. I tried several pharmaceutical pills that weren't "solving the problem."

After about one year of investigation, I felt that my body was at the mercy of doctors who did not see me as a whole person. They saw isolated symptoms that they could treat with pharmaceutical pills. They didn't care too much that many of the medications meant to be the "solution" were creating new health problems I hadn't had before this experiment began!

How was it that I felt sicker than before going to a doctor? Why didn't anyone care to ask me how I was doing emotionally? How did anyone expect to embrace healing if we continued seeing my body systems as separate entities? Why did the Western medical system leave me feeling so alone and unsupported?

I couldn't have understood this at the time, still indoctrinated under the treat-the-symptom system, disconnected from any holistic medicine practitioners. Yet, now I know that what triggered the flare-up of all of these digestive issues was trauma that I couldn't speak to because it felt too painful, and I felt deep shame.

When I was sixteen, I began to experience my first encounters with sexual assault, not having consented to a sexual situation, yet still watching it unfold within my own body. I felt such low self-worth at the time. Even though I knew it didn't feel right, I created stories to justify why I needed to continue living through these experiences. A huge part of me desired intimacy and connection, and I also felt an intense sexual curiosity. However, I couldn't put together that I was worthy of receiving these things without needing to lend my body in sexual ways that surpassed my limits. No one had taught me to speak to my authentic desires, mark boundaries, or give unambiguous yeses and nos.

I craved to express my confusion and shame with someone I could trust, but I felt that I couldn't think of any adult in my life who could handle receiving my experiences with care. I feared that if I told my mom, she would break down, swallowed by empathy and grief, and in an attempt to protect her, I couldn't find the courage to share something so painful. I also feared she would become extremely overprotective and prohibit me from attending parties and social gatherings. And early on in my life, I learned that my dad was not someone I could fully trust, so I would never have gone to him about this kind of thing. At this time, I needed a supportive community of other adults I could trust who weren't my parents. They say it takes a village to raise a child, and for me, in these moments of navigating trauma, I needed the support of a loving village, not cold doctors in white lab coats.

So, as the digestion difficulties prevailed for a year, I made a decision not founded on anything more than the strength of my intuition. I decided to stop seeing all doctors, refrain from taking all pills, and become autonomous over my health and well-being. I began researching herbal supplements to support digestion and noticed a general improvement. I made huge shifts in my diet and aimed to fuel my body with natural foods that would help me feel good. Also, I sat down to have various conversations with my mom. While at the time, I didn't yet dare to fully tell her about the sexual assaults I had been experiencing, it was clear that a substantial emotional component played a role in this physical pain in my gut.

My mom wrote down on a piece of paper, "Let Go of Your Shit," and we chuckled at how accurate this pun was. She told me to keep this message with me and use it as a helpful reminder to let go whenever I was holding on too strong and resisting the natural flow of energy already in movement. I noticed how easy it was to hold on to stories of anger, resentment, frustration, and feeling like the victim and how that story continued to reproduce in the life experiences I created. It seemed like a broken record playing out the same way, with different disguises each time. I began to develop labels about "the enemies," who mostly took the form of male-presenting individuals.

I was also still holding on to the pain of not being able to trust my dad. I reencountered that pain by finding myself in risky sexual situations with men I couldn't trust to care for me or respect my boundaries. I watched that same pain and distrust manifest in my male doctors, which I felt had left me more wounded than before. My digestive tract was trying so hard to hold on to my shit that it created pain and imbalance within my physical body. My emotional body was having difficulty letting go, forgiving, and moving on, and this pain continued to live within me.

Over the years, I noticed that my digestive issues mostly went away. At the onset of the flare-ups, my doctors gave me a chronic diagnosis, meaning I would be doomed to endure digestive problems throughout my life! Now, I have mainly noticed that I will only experience some acute flare-up when an emotional response directly triggers it.

And that brings me to today, ten years later, once again holding myself compassionately and lovingly as I witness myself experiencing considerable resistance to letting go. A challenging conversation occurred between me, my partner, and his friend, where I felt unworthy, attacked, threatened, and unsafe. While I know that neither my partner nor his friend intended to hurt me, I began to feel small and shut down during and after the conversation. My throat closed, and my muscles tensed, preventing me from sharing my empowered truth. My old patterning coping mechanisms led me to label the male bodies as enemies. This minor incident blew up within my body, and I began projecting my narratives onto this moment, witnessing anger and resentment bubble up to the surface.

After this conversation, I had horrible acid reflux for days and extremely anxious dreams. I felt that my body was regurgitating this event repeatedly, holding on to this story in which men took advantage of me. It has been over a week since the conversation, and I feel deeply humbled by how loving and forgiving my partner has been throughout this process. I am grateful for how he holds our diverse perspectives on this shared lived experience.

I see myself still holding on to so much judgment, disgust, and anger in the reflection of his open heart. I sense that he is calling me gently into a more easeful way where I can feel through and transmute my anger and resentment into forgiveness. I believe resentment is one of the most toxic human emotions, like drinking poison and expecting the other person to die. And each time that resentment winds its way into my emotional field, I feel called to remember a few important lessons. One is to accept others, a situation, an experience, just as it is and love it with compassion and understanding without needing to change anything about it. Another is to mark clear limits and boundaries from the beginning so I don't collapse later on, feeling stretched, worn, and drained. Another lesson is to fully express my rage in a safe container when it arises so that it doesn't remain trapped within me.

I believe rage is a sacred, powerful emotion that must be felt within our bodies. If we are one with nature's cycles, she too expresses her rage through devastating storms, crippling earthquakes, volcano eruptions, and endlessly dry droughts. As a woman, I was explicitly socialized never to express rage. Sure, I was more than welcome to express joy, beauty, and even sadness, but rage was prohibited. Rage was seen as something dangerous and inevitably violent. So, of course, simply because certain emotions were forbidden, I couldn't stop myself from feeling them. All the rage remained inside me, fermenting, yearning to be expressed, searching for an outlet, longing for fresh air.

So, what are safe and healthy ways to express emotions, specifically rage? We'll each have our coping mechanisms because each body is its own universe. Still, a few of my favorites include going for a run, primal screaming, rageful dancing, making music, and shaking. Find your safe container to express your rage and practice the courage to ask for what you need in those moments. Maybe you need to communicate to your housemates that you must scream and express wildly, like an electric storm, and when it's all over, you would like to cry into their arms, receive a loving touch, and drink a soothing cup of tea. Perhaps you want to share the story behind that emotion, and maybe you don't. It is entirely up to you if you would like to share. It is not your responsibility to fill others in on your process. Listen to and honor your body, allowing yourself to feel what needs to move through you.

I am grateful for this opportunity to see where my wounds and triggers are still alive in me, and I am reminded that I am free to transform and rewrite my story at any moment. I am premenstrual, on day 27 of my cycle, and I know this is the most potent time to let go and invite a fresh new beginning.

Me Entierro, I Bury Myself

"Me Entierro" — "I Bury Myself" — is a song I wrote in a moon blood ritual in Santiago de Chile. This particular moon blood ceremony was highly impactful because I had already purchased my ticket back home to California. It was a hot summer day in January 2020, and my body knew this would be my last moon cycle before immersing myself in a new phase of *mi camino*, my path. I was closing the chapter of an incredibly transformative three-year journey in South America and felt I had the space to reflect on all the growth I had embodied throughout this large cycle. So I sat by a beautiful tree in my friend's backyard, built a nature altar of flowers, leaves, sticks, and stones, and dug a small hole. I lit candles, burned palo santo, and set my obsidian and rose quartz yoni eggs on the altar.

Against the tree, I leaned my ukulele (the instrument that had been my partner for the last five years of my life and throughout my three-year journey). As I looked upon this work of art, I heard a loud call, deep within me, asking me to let go of my ukulele and gift it to my sister, who had been hosting me in her home. The thought of giving away my ukulele was terrifying and simultaneously liberating. I began to imagine the potential abundance that could continue to flow my way by creating space to receive new magic.

I had always wanted to play the guitar but felt it was too big and challenging. So, sticking with my ukulele created a sense of safety and comfort. I also imagined packing up my bags and heading to the next phase of my journey with my hands completely free and open to receiving. Since I always had my ukulele in hand, this would be the first time in the journey that I would have my hands free! So, with the thrilling, exciting energy of letting go and surrendering to the mystery, I poured my jar of moon blood onto the altar.

I then went to get my friend's guitar (not knowing many chords or even feeling confident in my guitar-playing abilities), and I began improvising with some of the thoughts and sensations flowing through me. I felt highly connected to the four elements and observed them moving through my being. I kept repeating this idea of burying myself.

My moon time is always an opportunity to return to my roots, ground myself, restore, and begin anew. And now, soon returning to the place of my birth after being away for so many years, I was experiencing this on a massive scale. I reflected on how seeds need those moments of darkness, stillness, and fertile soil beneath the surface to sprout and flourish in their own time. After constantly moving for so long, I started craving that sensation of stillness and rooting (all the while feeling frightened). Yet, just like the changing seasons and the constantly changing phases of the moon, I honored my decision and celebrated the transformation that would occur in the next cycle.

Below, you will find an English translation of the song and the original lyrics in Spanish.

I Bury Myself

I bury myself, I plant myself, I gift my moon to your clay
In the winter, I travel inward
In the spring and with the new moon, I am reborn again
I aliven myself, I am moving through spirals
From the darkness toward the light, expanding
Flourishing from my sacred womb space
Reclaiming my power, discovering deep pleasure
In your oceans, your mountains, your winds,
Your blazing fires flow in me
I am singing, awakening, and remembering
Offering the best version of me
Opening myself to receive, trusting in the mystery
The stars guide my flight, and the plants carry medicine
They teach me how to heal, inside I hear their song
In your oceans, your mountains, your winds,
Your blazing fires burn in me
Reclaiming my power
The power to be here, the power to create
The power to improvise the music that flows from inside
That shines from inside, that glows from inside
That is born from inside of me
From my sacred river, center of my power
She holds all of the memories
I clean my past, and I am reborn again
Here I begin to remember
Here I return to awaken
Right here, right now
I bury myself

Me Entierro

Me entierro, me siembro, entrego mi luna a tu arcilla
En el invierno marchito
En primavera y luna nueva vuelvo a renacer
Me avivo, espiralando ando
Desde la oscuridad, hacia la luz y más allá
Floreciendo, desde mi vientre sagrado
Recobrando mi poder, descubriendo el placer
En tus mares, tus montañas, tus vientos
Tus incendios fluyen en mi
Voy cantando, despertando, y recordando
Ofrendando lo mejor de mi
Abriéndome a recibir, confiando en el misterio
Las estrellas guían mi vuelo y las plantas llevan medicina
Me enseñan a curar, adentro escucho su cantar
En tus mares, tus montañas, tus vientos
Tus incendios arden en mi
Recobrando mi poder
Poder estar aquí, poder crear
Poder improvisar la música
Que fluye desde adentro, que brilla desde adentro
Que nace desde adentro de mi
De mi río sagrado, centro del poder
Guarda la memoria de todo el ayer
Limpio mi pasado, vuelvo a renacer
Aquí comienzo a recordar
Aquí comienzo a despertar
Aqui ahora
Me entierro

Triggered Face Down

In August 2021, I was making love with my partner of one year. We both felt extremely sensitive, as if our capacity to tune into the diverse expressions of pleasure was hyper-aware. As we rolled through waves of delicious sensations within our bodies, we ended up in a new position in which I was lying flat on my belly, and he was penetrating me from behind, placing his entire body weight on me. Suddenly, I switched from a place of trust, love, safety, and surrender to a state of panic. "This is the exact position I was raped in years ago," I thought. I tried to bring myself back into the present moment and remind myself that I was not trapped. I was consenting to this sexual exchange. Additionally, I told myself I had the opportunity to reclaim this position by creating new embodied cellular memories of pleasure and love where pain, fear, and numbness once existed. Although I used my mind to come up with reasons why I should be okay with this, I began to feel tears stream down my cheeks, and that is when I asked for a pause.

My partner moved off of me, and we lay beside each other, breathing heavily. The tears continued to roll down slowly, and I felt my partner look at me with curiosity and compassion. His eyes held me in a softness that invited me to share what was happening without a rush to tell a story. I felt pretty speechless, as if my words were buried in layers deep within myself. So I managed to say something like, "I am okay…. Give me a minute…. Thank you for your patience." After I felt collected enough to speak about what had come up for me, I asked him if he would be willing to hear a story, to which he responded with a clear yes.

I flashed back five years before when I studied abroad in Quito, Ecuador. I remember having a group of male friends who were musicians. Since I was new to the city, I enjoyed having artist friends who could connect me with the local music scene. From my first encounter with these men, I felt a strong presence of machismo and dark, deep pain within them that they often masked with massive amounts of alcohol.

I was at a live music party in an abandoned house with these men and many others. We began drinking together, and I somehow made out with Miguel. Miguel led me into a makeshift room with giant empty window frames and no doors. So, in a sense, there was not much seclusion or privacy. He pushed me against a wall and started kissing me. I felt nervousness in my belly that I couldn't speak to. I was reminded of when I was pushed against a wall at age eighteen by this guy I had a huge crush on for a while. Yes, there was some attraction and desire to explore intimacy, but at the time, things were moving faster than I was comfortable with.

Eighteen-year-old me fell onto my knees as he pushed my shoulders down and shoved his cock into my mouth. Eighteen-year-old me kneeled paralyzed as he fucked my mouth, came, zipped up his pants, and then walked away.

So here I was with Miguel as he kept grabbing my hand to touch his penis, and I kept pushing my hand away, telling him that I did not want to touch his penis. He didn't seem to hear me because he kept grabbing my hand, and although I said no, I also kind of giggled as I said it, so perhaps he interpreted it as a playful no, even though I meant to express a stern no. I felt guilty giving my no, as if I owed him something. So perhaps as I gave my no, I said it playfully and kindly so that he would accept me.

Was my sense of self-worth so fragile that I needed the validation of a man who wouldn't respect my boundaries? Why was I so concerned about being rejected by a man who made me feel unsafe? Although we only communicated in Spanish, he asked me in English, "Do you know how to suck dick?" And I responded in Spanish, "Yes, I do," once again in a lighthearted tone and playfully rolling my eyes, seeming slightly annoyed. And he said, again in English, "Prove it." I began to feel frustrated, disgusted, and unsafe since I got the message that he was not hearing me and was only invested in his pleasure. Yet I also thought that it was somehow my responsibility to give him the sexual pleasure he desired, even if I didn't desire it. Luckily, I told him I just wanted to return to the party, and although he seemed frustrated and disappointed, he accepted it.

After that night, I didn't feel like my consent had been violated or that I would never engage with this man sexually again. I still felt kind of curious about exploring sexual intimacy together. So when he asked if I was interested in hanging out a few days later, I said yes. I arrived at a park at night where Miguel and a handful of other men were already extremely drunk. As soon as I arrived, I felt a bit of fear and compromised safety, and perhaps the men sensed this in me, so they offered me a lot of alcohol, incessant amounts, as they kept telling me to lighten up. Soon, I was completely drunk.

Naturally, Miguel and I started making out again, and I felt super incapable of marking any clear limits or boundaries due to how intoxicated I felt. I knew I needed to get home because I felt drunk and unsafe at night in a park in the middle of the city, surrounded only by men. I must have asked one of the men to support me in getting a taxi home because the next thing I knew, a taxi had pulled up. Miguel and I had gotten in the back together, making out drunkenly and sloppily. I hadn't even given the taxi driver the directions to my house, and suddenly, I realized we had arrived at Miguel's house. He told me to come inside.

When we walked in, his parents were sitting in the living room watching T.V. I ran straight to the bathroom to throw up. I felt so unbelievably drunk that after my purge, I walked into Miguel's room and plopped my dizzy body onto the bed facedown. He came in from behind me and started whispering in my ear that he wanted to have sex with me, to which I responded, "Not now," because I only felt half-conscious. Then he pulled down my pants from behind and slipped his penis into my vagina as he poured his entire body weight onto me in a way that completely pinned me down.

Perhaps I could have had the tools to escape that violent situation if I hadn't been so intoxicated. Still, at the moment, the only response my body had was paralysis. I completely shut down in stillness and shock that this was happening to me. I felt his thrusts so painful inside of me that a few times, I cried out, "Oww!" He responded by covering my mouth and telling me to be quiet. After all, his parents were in the room next door in this tiny apartment, and he probably wanted to keep the fact that he was raping me on the down low. I felt a part of me was still in my body, feeling the painful physical sensations. And a huge part of me had left my body, like witnessing this traumatic scene from above.

Suddenly, I felt him pull off of me, and I felt wetness between my legs. There was cum in my vagina, and I asked him if he had cummed inside me, which he did, but he didn't look me in the eyes. He just grabbed my shoes, slipped them on my feet, and told me that the taxi was waiting outside for me to take me home. I felt like a robot simply moving through motions. Speechless, I grabbed my things and walked past his parents in the living room, who said goodnight to me. I walked outside and got in the taxi home.

I tried to process what had occurred but couldn't think clearly. I couldn't hold space for the emotional impact this had on me. At least I still had an IUD then, so I didn't have to worry about pregnancy, but I was worried about STDs. In the coming weeks, I pretended that nothing had happened and took an STD test, which returned negative.

As I told this story and wrote it, I cried, feeling how painful that traumatic event was and how alone I felt in moving through it. It took me months to claim that this experience was a sexual assault and hold space for the pain present within my body, love it, and transform it. I am infinitely grateful to my partner for holding a compassionate space for me to share this story. Witnessing trauma arising in a pleasurable, loving, and consensual encounter was challenging. I initially felt frustrated. "Why do such painful memories need to live in the same place of my body, home to creation and sexual pleasure?" And I know these wounded parts of me will not transform through frustration. They surface to remind me that they are part of my narrative. They ask to be seen, acknowledged, and held in love. And they ask to be given the space to grieve or rage or feel what I may need to feel now since, for so long, I only felt numbness. As I hold myself gently, I remember that this process is slow and delicate and that every lived experience is another opportunity for more profound healing and growth.

Rejected by a Could-Be Lover

This Fall of 2020, I have taken a Thanksgiving road trip with a could-be lover down the Mexican Coast. I am sitting in a little cave on the ocean's edge in Baja California, Mexico. I just built an altar of rocks, shells, and seaweed and poured out my menstrual blood to offer to the mother ocean. Now, I feel calm, free, full, and grateful.

I am also feeling frustrated as I question, "Why is mutual, turned-on, let-me-pleasure-you, fully surrendered attraction so difficult to come by?" Maybe in general or maybe just for me, but I have been reflecting on the numerous times in my life that I was with a man, and they were turned on and sexually wanted me. Yet, I was so unattracted, disgusted, and utterly uninterested in engaging sexually with them.

And often, I explicitly said no, but that no wasn't respected. After so many times of saying no and feeling exhausted from keeping my guard up, instead of walking away, I let them follow through with their sexual fantasy. Even though I had not consented and was not engaged, I allowed these men to use my body as a hole for their pleasure.

And then I thought about so many times that I was fully tuned into my pleasure state, ready to give and receive the brightest light within me like, "Hey baby, are you ready to play and create right here and now, elevating our spirits and bodies in a pleasurable, consensual, loving way?" And I received a 'no' many times, which I completely respected and accepted. I feel frustrated that I wasn't heard or respected when I gave my "no," yet when I felt turned on and present, and my body said "TOTAL, YES," when I received a no, I fully honored it.

Maybe the key is to continue the conversation after the "no" and have both individuals verbally communicate what they are uncomfortable with in the present moment. Yet continuing to be vulnerable after receiving a "no" can be challenging because as soon as I hear a "no," my body may shut down and feel too rejected to continue exploring intimacy. When my body goes into rejection mode, I often feel my toes curl, my muscles tense, my heartbeat quicken, and an overwhelming need to escape. My rejection response urges me to find safety, love, and comfort as if my survival depended on it. It has been helpful for me to recognize my body's response to feelings of rejection so that I may be a witness to the shifts in my nervous system and assure myself that I am, in fact, safe and unthreatened.

A few weeks before this Thanksgiving road trip, a could-be-lover came to my home for a planned sleepover. We had only had one sexual exchange before, so I was curious about the potential for some form of intimacy to continue unfolding between us. We had a sweet night cooking dinner and hiking in the desert rocky mountains behind my home, but his energy was standoffish and distant, and he even asked to sleep in a separate bed. I felt deeply rejected and didn't feel it was safe to express what was happening. I feared he might judge or deny my lived experience and then reject me for sharing my whole self. I had expected that if we were going to have a sleepover, we would be open to exploring intimacy together. I had no sexual expectations but a desire to share tender space. I wasn't just offering him a bed in a hostel. I was opening up an opportunity for us to spend quality time together.

Ultimately, he went to sleep pretty early in the bed next to mine without even saying goodnight. I went up to my room to find him asleep, snoring loudly. I felt so hurt, unconsidered, and disgusted in that moment. I felt I needed to crawl into child's pose, cry, and be held lovingly. I would have loved my feelings of rejection to have been witnessed and received a compassionate, non-judgmental touch, holding space for me to move through my process. I was too embarrassed to confess how much I had felt him rejecting me and pushing me away. How could I continue investing energy in a man demonstrating that he was emotionally unavailable? I felt such an uncomfortable sadness because it wasn't just him. He symbolized and triggered within me so many past experiences of not belonging and specifically being rejected by men. Here was my wounded self showing up to repeat a pattern that felt comfortable, familiar, and inevitably hurtful to me.

From a young age, I felt disconnected from my father. He was often emotionally unavailable, disinterested, and unsupportive. My mother and father were the first humans I interacted with upon arriving on this Earth, and these relationships became imprinted in my cellular memory. Although I had supposedly done my part to heal these relationships, a part of my subconscious constantly craved what it knew as a child, however toxic it may have been.

So, in this scenario, I saw the roles play out so clearly. I felt like a little girl saying, "Hey, Dad, do you want to play with me?" And this could-be-lover responded in such a way, barely using words, but simply with nonverbal cues that indicated, "Can't you see that I am unavailable? Leave me alone!" I felt compassion for these men's wounds because I knew that deep down, a father wants to play with his daughter and support and nurture her even if he doesn't know how. And this could-be-lover also desired to create intimacy in some way. Otherwise, why would he have agreed to sleep over at my home? There is a little boy inside these men who also yearns to be loved and held, but lifetimes of protective mechanisms make it extremely challenging to be vulnerable and move directly toward what feels good. These unhealed wounds and unmet needs often reproduce suffering for themselves and others.

So here I am, Mother Ocean, witnessing the layers of armor inside of me and inside of this man. The present dynamic is beyond awkward because we have driven down to Mexico together, and I have been unable to express how I feel impacted by his distance and lack of communication. And here we are, camping together but sleeping in separate tents, somehow pretending that nothing sexual ever occurred between us.

When did we forget how beautiful and healing it is to surrender to each other fully?

When did we forget that we all deserve uplifting, safe, pleasurable love?

With this moon blood, I allow my relationships to transform, accept and honor my boundaries, release what no longer serves me, and trust in the tides as I dance with the ebbs and flows of these cyclical waves.

Healing the Father Wound

I am in San Agustin, Colombia, one year into my backpacking journey. I came into town yesterday after being deep in the mountains for the last few weeks. Most of the people staying at the hostel are "brothers and sisters" I had met in a peaceful rainbow community, so I was shocked when the hostel turned into a wild, uncontrolled party last night.

The night began with a relaxed communal energy, but soon, everyone around me got unbelievably drunk, and many were taking various drugs. The energy turned dark, and I felt unsafe. I danced a bit, trying to enjoy myself, but ultimately, I just fell asleep in the bed I was sharing with my friend. (Since you paid per bed at this hostel, not per person, my friends and I teamed up, and six of us shared a room with three beds). I heard the party until late, and I half slept until the sun began to rise.

Suddenly, I awoke because I felt a hand moving over my butt and vagina. I turned to look at my friend, certain he was touching me. We had never engaged in any sexual way, and I fully trusted that he would never touch my genitals without consent. I looked at his face and found him sleeping deeply. I saw both of his hands snuggled into his pillow. I tried to turn around and go back to sleep, thinking that perhaps it was just a ghost sensation, but a few seconds later, I felt the hand touch me again. So I sat up quickly and pushed the covers off to see what was happening, and I discovered a local man hiding under the bed touching me. I began screaming at him, "What are you doing?" He got up and moved clumsily toward the door. Since he was beyond drunk, he couldn't run far and only managed to stumble slowly into the hallway. With this, everyone in the room awoke.

Immediately, I began to cry. "*Otra vez*," I thought, "Again?" My body was shocked. Although the moment of violation was painful, it was much more painful to deal with everyone's reactions. The first responses from my friends in the room assured me that I had only woken up from a bad dream and that this did not happen in real life. Then, people asked me if I had been at the party and had gotten drunk and why I had even left the door open in the first place. These questions directly blamed me as everyone tried to understand from a place of logic instead of supporting me from a heart space. And then some converted this into their drama. They would tell me angrily that this was sexual abuse and that I had to tell the police, and they proceeded to tell my story to everyone who entered the hostel that day. Suddenly, my private and personal story became everyone else's story. No one asked for my consent to share this story. No one asked me what I needed or how they could best support me. They just told everyone that Aviva had been the victim of abuse.

That day, I prayed to the Great Spirit and asked for support to heal my body and wounds. I asked to reconnect to my inner strength. I asked to understand what was inside me that kept attracting sexual abuse and violation of my body.

What wound do I have yet to embrace in love, transform, and release so I can cease to repeat this same lived experience?

As I carried these reflections with me throughout the day, I connected with a mother of the mountain community who was also in town, and she held space to support me and hear my story. I feared my life would be a never-ending list of sexual assaults. She shared that she, too, was a survivor of sexual abuse and that she had healed this wound through regression therapy. She offered to support me by diving into my subconscious and exploring what wound was unhealed inside of me that led me to repeat this pattern, without victim blaming myself but taking ownership of my healing journey and acknowledging my wounds within.

I felt hesitant. After all, I would need to return to the mountain, a place I had eagerly left because I had developed a worsening staphylococcus infection. I felt I needed to take care of my physical body before immersing myself in more profound spiritual and emotional healing. I felt it would be irresponsible to spend all my energy in the spirit realm processing emotional trauma. In contrast, my physical body, the temple of my spirit, had a serious infection that worsened each day. If I continued to neglect the health of my physical body, then my spirit would have nowhere to return.

While I typically turn to natural herbal medicines 99% of the time, this seemed like an emergency, and I felt I needed the support of Western antibiotics. This woman insisted that her medicine would benefit me and that I could cure my infection by sending it love and squeezing fresh lemon juice on my wounds. While I felt uncertain about which step to take, I also felt alone and vulnerable and nourished by the possibility of receiving support from a mother who seemed to be offering her medicine out of the goodness of her heart. So I agreed to follow this woman guardian angel back up the mountain. Antibiotics would have to wait.

At the first regression, two men were present as her supporters in case she became too triggered by what we discovered. We began by lighting candles, setting intentions, and calling upon the angels to accompany this journey. I remember they asked me if I needed anything before diving into the regression, and I felt so exposed and cornered—like I couldn't fully trust them to ask for what I needed. How was I supposed to let these humans witness my subconscious if I couldn't even claim my needs to them in waking life? If I could have asked for something then, I probably would have asked if each of them could put a hand on my back while I wept in a child's pose. Instead, I just said that I needed nothing, and I blindfolded myself to begin.

As she guided me to visualize a path, I walked down, down, down, and eventually arrived at a door. Here, I was asked to grab paint and a brush and write the topic of this regression on the door. I chose red paint and wrote *"Violaciones Sexuales* – Sexual Abuse." Walking through the door, I found darkness with nothing to orient me. So I was guided to ask someone for help, perhaps my dad. Although I strongly resisted asking my dad for support at that moment, they encouraged me to speak to him. I had to explain to my dad's spirit where I was and what I was doing, and I asked if he would be willing to help me. Of course, he said no. Like always, I felt disappointed by his emotional unavailability. However, the facilitators encouraged me to ask him what he needed to be able to support me. He said that he needed a hug. My body felt stiff and tense. I did not want to hug him, even in the spirit realm. We asked him who he needed a hug from, and he said his mother. So then we had to call upon his mother, a grandmother who left this Earth before I joined it. I presented myself as her granddaughter and asked if she could support me in this regression, to which she responded with a yes. The regression went on for several hours, so without going into infinite detail about the process, we harvested incredible jewels from this exploration.

We could see my father's wounds and the sadness he carried from having emotionally unavailable parents. His inner child was never given the care and nurture he craved, so as an adult, he had no idea how to be a fully present father. Throughout the session, I felt frustrated, like, "Why are we still talking about my father? Can he please go away now so I can get to the root of this sexual abuse problem?"

The facilitators encouraged me to stick with what was arising because everything we discovered about my relationship with my father was a beautiful reflection of the toxic ways I had been engaging with other men throughout my life. It was interesting to notice the frustration and resistance toward my father shift throughout the session. I was encouraged to practice compassion and forgiveness toward him and send him waves of gratitude for showing up in the best way he knew.

When I emerged from the session, I felt much lighter and relieved. I felt I had done my part to transform many internal puzzle pieces, but I questioned how to integrate all this information into my waking life. The proposal was to hold a series of regressions throughout a few weeks in which we would continue to explore this topic of sexual abuse and gain practical tools for my healing. However, my staph infection worsened after about a week, and I had to leave the mountainous jungle. I needed soap, clean water, and antibiotics, things that this community could no longer support me with. So, although I would have wanted to continue this regression therapy, I left one early morning before sunrise straight into the town's medical center.

Naturally, my staph infection healed after a few weeks, and I began reaching out more to my dad through phone calls. Unfortunately, the calls were typically short and unfulfilling. I usually felt hurt that one of the two humans who brought me onto this Earth knew me superficially. I learned to make peace with our phone calls, releasing any expectations that he would profoundly support me and simply surrendering to the conversation that he could offer me in the present moment. This relationship is one that I can never say, "Tada! Fully healed!" and wrap the bow neatly on top. It's constantly rising to the surface and asking to be seen.

I have learned a lot about marking clear boundaries, acceptance, forgiveness, and how much space is safe and necessary within a relationship. I can't point the finger at him and blame him for how I was traumatized by our relationship. Instead, I can feel gratitude for having the inner strength to visit these wounded and traumatized parts of me, hold them in love, and transform them. After all, they say that we choose our parents, so it is for a reason that I was called to Earth as his daughter.

May we all continue to have the courage to transform the wounds we carry within. For our parents, grandparents, and ancestors who didn't have the support and resources they needed to heal. May we shed, release, and transform for our children, our lineage, and all of humanity yet to come.

Slowing Down Into the Darkness

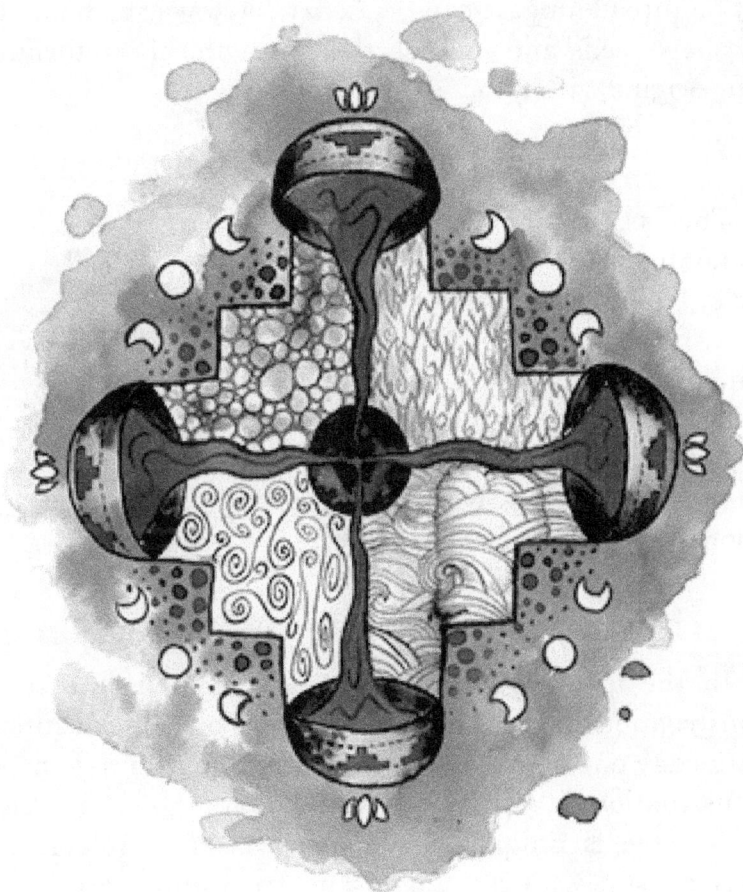

Moon's Energy

With the darkness of the new moon (approximately days 1-7 of the moon cycle), this is a powerful time to slow down, travel inward, and protect your energy from external influences. You may experience heightened sensitivity as your inner shadow self comes out to greet you. This darkness need not be threatening. It can be a cozy, safe, warm container to sew new seeds and nourish their growth, like returning to your origins within the womb.

Moon Phase: New Moon

This is the time of the New Moon, containing the darkest nights of this cycle. Hold space to be with the dark skies. Take an evening stroll within your internal cosmos. Lie out to gaze at the vast heavens. You may discover some hidden gems in the darkness. After all, the nights with the darkest moon also hold the starriest skies.

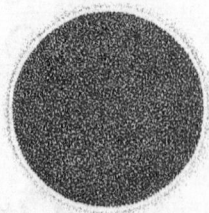

Menstrual Cycle Phase: Menstruation

In the menstrual cycle, the new moon is the time of menstruation. Whenever the first day of bleeding occurs, this marks day one of a brand new moon cycle within your body. Menstruation is a powerful time for your body to release. Each cycle is unique, so you may need to release grief, trauma, pain, sadness, anger, and frustration in one cycle. Perhaps you may release gratitude, celebration, forgiveness, and joy in the next cycle. Throughout your cycle, your body has been cultivating a nourishing home in your uterus, lining the walls with the most fertile life force energy to sustain the birthing of a new life. Assuming your body has sunk into the destruction mode of tearing down the uterine lining in the premenstrual phase, in the menstrual phase, your uterus opens and begins to release this blood.

In a way, I feel that my menstrual blood is an invitation to shed and let go of all that no longer serves me and also to revisit memories that have been stored inside of my uterus (in my previous cycles, throughout my lifetime, and even stretching back to past generational trauma and wisdom). It is also an invitation to get a closer look at what is happening in my inner world. Each cycle, I form a deeper relationship with my blood by observing its color, smell, texture, quantity, consistency, etc., and by learning more about my menstrual blood, I learn more about myself as a whole being.

In my experience tracking my cycles, it has been a nourishing practice for me to bring awareness and compassion to the sensations I may be experiencing during my bleed. By acknowledging these menstrual patterns, I have cultivated a more profound sense of trust in myself to meet my needs in this magical phase. With every cycle, I discover more about caring for my bleeding self. I typically feel low energy, lethargic, irritable, bloated, needing silence, withdrawn, slow-paced, and calm. This is when I only have enough energy and desire to care for myself. Anything that I usually would be excited to tend to in any other moment of my cycle may seem exhausting and impossible to achieve in my moon time. I can feel overcome with a sensation that my womb is a portal to bleed the world's pain, and I need to curl up into my bed and allow myself to cry. I do not like to feel that my boundaries are stretched or tested in this phase. I feel most open to receiving support from others during this time and being nurtured by my community. I may crave a massage from a loved one, a warm and yummy cooked meal, or even a simple cup of tea.

There are infinite overlapping spirals within your body that send messages and indicators about your overall health. Some practices can diagnose disease and imbalances within the body by using the ears, feet, eyes, or tongue to map the holistic picture within your body. The womb is one of those mandalas as well. It is the defining sacred center of your body, mind, and spirit. The health of your womb is a reflection of your overall health, and your menstrual blood is a beautiful opportunity to peek at what is going on in your inner world.

Surrendering and opening to receiving has been highly challenging for me (since I typically feel most empowered when I am in my action-oriented independent ovulation phase.) So, nurturing myself with softness in the menstrual phase is a beautiful reminder to slow down, rest, recharge, and ask for help. It is my most vulnerable time of the month because I have to ask for support to fulfill specific responsibilities, and I must trust that I have woven a web for myself and my community where all bleeding bodies are genuinely invited and encouraged to make any adjustments they may need throughout their moon time. For me, menstruation is a meditation in which I can release all of the expectations that I typically place upon myself and hold space for my process, keeping my faith that everything will be okay even if I need to retreat for a few days.

If it is available to you in these days of menstruation, see if you can pause daily work, take a long warm bath, and practice asking for what you desire. This is a beautiful time to write out intentions for the cycle, reflect on the past cycle, and nurture these new seeds with care so that you may harvest them in the upcoming full moon (ovulation time). The more you give yourself permission to rest and recharge during this time, the more you can blossom into your fully fertile, juicy self in ovulation. Allow yourself to surrender to the waves and dance fully with your flow.

Since your womb and energetic fields are completely open at this time, it is crucial to discern what energies you are letting in. Be selective about your conversations, the space you hold for others, and the people you may or may not want to be around. An excellent way to protect your womb space is to tie a red yarn around your waist and keep it on throughout your bleed days. As a witchy act of self-love and creative expression, you can make space to weave your waist protection with yarn, a special scarf, beads, crystals, and some medicinal herbs. Get creative about ways that you can protect your center and keep this area warm and cozy.

There are many different ways to release and capture your blood during menstruation. I strongly suggest that you refrain from using tampons and disposable pads. Not only are they extraordinarily wasteful and disastrous for Mother Earth, but they are also full of toxic chemicals that disrupt hormones. These products carry carcinogens, bleach, and even pesticides that can bring sickness to your womb. Instead, I will offer a few suggestions you can explore in your bleed time and alternate throughout your moon, depending on your needs. Find a method that works with your flow as it flows. Since it constantly changes, you may need different things each cycle and at different moments in your bleeding days.

For a long time, I loved my reusable menstrual cup. It is easy to wash. It is simple to collect my blood and transfer it into a glass jar for an offering or painting. It is pretty comfortable. I never really feel it inside of me. It lasts for up to five years. In many ways, I think the reusable menstrual cup was a perfect way for me to ease back into bleeding since I had previously used tampons. This was like a healthy, eco-friendly version of a tampon. As soon as I realized that I was essentially using a different version of a tampon, I stopped loving the cup. The cup creates a lot of suction within the vaginal canal and sexual organs. It is essentially like putting a cork in place within my body that wants to release and flow freely. It is easier to forget that I am bleeding when I have my cup in because I don't feel the blood fully flowing out of me. I also tend to feel more cramps when I have my cup in. Sometimes, putting my cup in and focusing on other things feels supportive. But if it works with my flow, I mostly avoid my menstrual cup.

I resonate most with reusable menstrual pads and menstrual underwear. This is a slower option because washing blood from a cloth requires more effort than rinsing a menstrual cup. But this is a part of the beauty of the process since, after all, my moon time is a gift for me in which I am allowed to slow down. I appreciate this option because I can feel the blood fully flowing out of me. I can smell her and interact with her color and texture. I feel that I am not damming the flow as I allow the blood to flow out of me entirely.

Turning these bloody cloths into an opportunity for a moon blood offering is pretty simple. After I have bled in my menstrual underwear or cloth, I place this cloth in a small bucket of cold water. I typically allow these cloths to soak for a few hours or overnight. Then, upon returning, I find beautifully tinted red water prepared to share with the plants in my garden or to pour out as an offering on my moon blood altar.

There is always an option to free bleed. This can look like placing a towel out under the sun and relaxing naked as you write in your journal, meditate, sing, and create art. As your blood releases from your womb, there is absolutely nothing that detains her. She flows where she would like to go. Perhaps she flows straight back to Mother Earth as you pee. Maybe she gets messy between your legs, and you rinse her off in a warm shower later. Perhaps as she flows out of you, you paint directly with this blood straight from your womb onto a canvas. You can even free-bleed by wearing a long skirt and nothing else underneath as you move through your day. Of course, this option works best if you are in a safe, comfortable home environment and you feel the courage and curiosity to allow your blood to flow as you release any feelings of shame, embarrassment, and disgust about her. Some bleeding bodies can feel their blood beginning to flow, so they contract their sexual organs and then only release their blood actively and consciously when they pee.

There are many ways to collect and offer your moon blood, including several I haven't named. So, in your next menstruation, explore practices and rituals that feel meaningful, witchy, and nourishing. Whether you dilute your moon blood in water and offer it to your plants as a fertilizer, paint your own body, a canvas, or on paper, hold a moon planting ritual by building a nature altar and returning your blood to Mother Earth as a love offering, create your version of a Red Tent and call upon your sisters, trust in your moon blood, and connect with her in your intentional way.

Cervical Dance

As your cervix opens during menstruation, you shed fluids from your uterine lining. Pay attention to how dark or light the color of your blood is and how there are subtle shifts throughout your bleeding days. Pay attention to how thick or thin your blood is and see if you can connect to any particular emotions or memories you release. Typically, if you are shedding brown blood, this is a sign that your body has been holding on to something for too long, and you are now shedding old blood. If your blood is bright red, this typically is a sign of a freshly rejuvenated womb that is shedding what she has accumulated in the last cycle. If you find thick clots or any other "abnormalities," get curious about the messages that your body is trying to send you through your womb. During your bleed, your cervix will be in a firm low position.

Season: Winter

This is the season of the cold winter and hibernation. In the wintertime, the days are short, and the nights are long, creating a supportive cocoon for us to travel inward. After the land has given us abundant harvests through the Spring, Summer, and Fall, this is the time to rest and snuggle up by the fire.

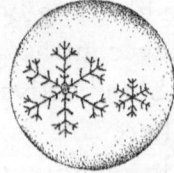

Element: Water

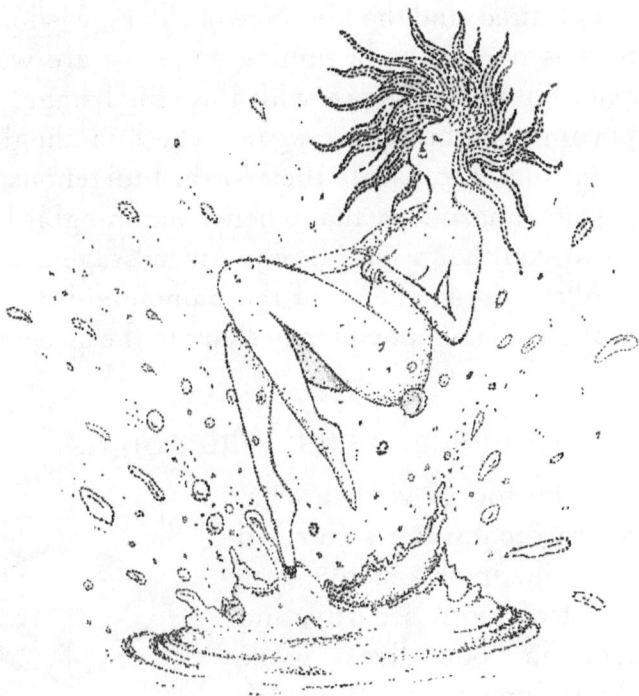

This is the element of water in which we may remember to flow without resistance. Water will always continue its flow through, above, below, or around something. There is nothing that can detain its natural course. So, as your womb opens up to flow, release any dams within your body and allow the emotions to pour freely. Rejuvenate yourself with herbal teas and floral baths, and hold space to pray with the water. May you have the courage to dive into your darkest oceans and dance freely in the light of your most transparent crystalline waters.

Direction: North

The direction is of the North, represented by the color white, the nighttime, and the life stage of elders, wisdom, and death. There is no end or beginning since we are working with a circle. So we can dance with this "final stage" of life as an opportunity to be reborn again. The hummingbird, a symbol of wisdom, represents the North. Indigenous tribes in the Peruvian Amazon say that when a hummingbird visits, this signals to you that a wise teacher or message is coming your way. Allow the medicine of the hummingbird to open your heart and soul so that you may share in the sweet nectar of life.

Astrological Signs: Water Signs

Cancer: The fourth Zodiac sign, Cancer, is a cardinal water sign ruled by the moon. She invites us to create a container of comfort, security, and nourishment in our lives while creating safe boundaries. Cancer's energy embodies the mother, the womb space, creating a membrane to differentiate what is safe to come into our intimate space and what must be put out. This is a powerful portal to reflect on your home, your family, and your community, as well as your sense of self within these spaces.

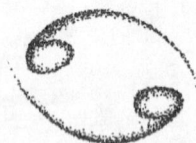

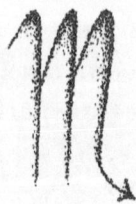

Scorpio: Scorpio is the eighth sign of the Zodiac, the second water sign, with a fixed quality. Scorpio's energy is intense as a water sign ruled by both Pluto and the fiery energy of Mars. This is a powerful portal for death and rebirth, bringing your shadow self out to dance in the light. Create a safe container to explore mysticism, sex, death, and pleasure taboos. Seek balance by dancing in the dark without getting sucked too deeply into cynism or depression.

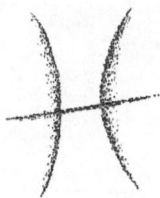

Pisces: Pisces is the twelfth sign of the Zodiac, the third and final water sign ruled by Jupiter, with a mutable quality. Pisces is an extremely emotional sign inviting a deeper connection with your dreams, spirituality, fantasy, and your deepest inner feelings. Pisces energy can dissolve and melt into its surroundings, losing one's sense of self. Create a container for creativity, imagination, and intuition, and allow your most whimsical self to pour through you. Be mindful of who and what is in your surroundings since, in this sensitivity, your center may merge with external influences.

Female Archetype:
Wise Old Woman & Grandmother

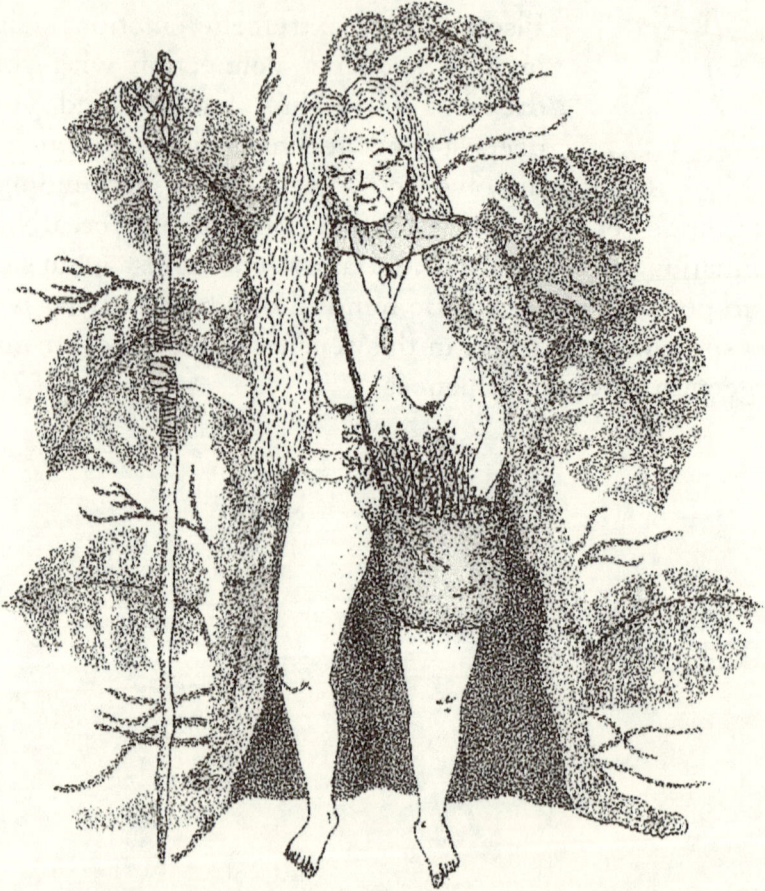

You may envision a wise old woman and grandmother archetype in this phase. This woman is also referred to as the Crone. The grandmother moves slowly, possessing infinite wisdom through lived experience. It is said that the uterus is the true heart center of a bleeding person, and in this moment of opening and releasing, you have access to endless wisdom and memories. Don't fear the expansive medicine you may witness within yourself during this time. Create space for yourself to tap into this embodied knowledge unapologetically. You'll be surprised what may channel through you in this receptive state. Elevate your prayers as you work with the thin veil of the spirit realm. You are never alone, and may your bleed time be a reminder of all the seen and unseen forces cheering you on and accompanying your growth. Perhaps in your lineage, your grandmother and mother were never allowed to slow down in their moon time and honor their bleeding body. Allow yourself to connect to your blood for healing and feel how it ripples infinitely outward, healing your ancestors and the ones yet to come.

Suggested Foods

Since you are shedding blood at this time, it is vital to replenish your body with nutrient-rich foods, especially those rich in iron. Great foods to incorporate during your moon time are lentils, kale, and all kinds of leafy greens. You can try making a veggie soup with warming herbs to stoke the fire within your womb. To support feeling grounded, you may want to incorporate root vegetables like carrots, onions, garlic, beets, sweet potatoes, ginger, and turmeric. Foods high in omega-3, like flax seeds and eggs, will support your body by reducing inflammation. In your bleed time, your reproductive hormones are at an all-time low, so listen to and honor the pace of your body. Perhaps you feel called to cleanse and incorporate some light fasting during a portion of your menstruation. Just be sure to replenish your body with plenty of fluids, and if you do feel called to eat hearty meals, aim for nutrient-dense foods. You may not have the energy to cook elaborate meals at this time, so you can always plan. Perhaps you know you will begin bleeding the next day, so you prepare a large batch of soup the night before and stick it in the fridge. You can also allow your loved ones to practice their generosity and ask them for the food they can prepare for you during your bleed time.

In my experience, it is helpful to avoid citrus on my moon days, as well as caffeinated drinks. I also avoid immersing my body in cold water. I have found that these things cause cramping during my bleeding, so I aim to nourish my body with a warming, soothing quality. There is no set formula for what may be a clear yes or no during menstruation. All bodies are different, and by tracking your cycle, you can gain more clarity on what feels most supportive to you.

Suggested Movement Plan

Movement is medicine, and it can be powerful medicine to discern when to surrender into stillness. It can be tempting to lie in bed all day, especially on heavy days of bleeding. If this is what your body is calling for, honor her and give her the much-needed rest she is asking for. If you are surrendering to complete rest, make sure to do so intentionally. Instead of lying in bed and watching television shows on your computer, see if you can use this moment of stillness to have a conversation with your womb, meditate with her, and feel her consciously releasing her blood. Don't be discouraged if you try to tune into your womb but feel an emptiness or an inability to listen to her. Each time you make the intention to feel and hear her, you will strengthen your capacity to tune into the messages of your womb. If you feel that you have it in you to incorporate some light movement, I strongly recommend this. Just by doing some light stretching, Yin yoga, chi gong, taking a lap around the block, or wiggling out to a few of your favorite songs, you will begin to produce endorphins that can soothe any menstrual pain, and you will increase blood flow throughout your body to support the releasing process.

Suggested Herbal Support

For further support in easing the release of menstrual blood, try to nurture your womb space with warmth. You may enjoy placing a heating pad on your belly and lying down. Try working with tummy-taming soothing herbs like Chamomile, Calendula, Lemon Balm, and Lavender. Also, anti-inflammatories like Ginger and Turmeric can ease menstrual cramps. Any suggested herbs can be taken as an oil, tincture, or tea, or you may want to sprinkle some fresh herbs into a warm bath.

Cyclical Gardening

Since a plant's waters have traveled down to the roots, most of its power lies below the surface. This is an excellent time to plant roots like potatoes, ginger, turmeric, etc., and also an ideal time to harvest roots since most of their medicine and nutrients are concentrated in their roots. It is also a good time to prune plants since their integrity is in their roots, and they will not suffer from shedding their leaves. While the roots are strong, you can clear away all of the extra foliage that can be shed to support the rejuvenation of the plant. Take it slow in your garden during this new moon time. Just as your body rests in menstruation, allow your garden to relax.

Writing Reflections

❭ What pleasure practice can you cultivate during menstruation that would feel good and nourishing?

❭ What do you need to feel safe to ask for the support you desire in this phase?

❭ Are you experiencing any resistance in sinking into a deeper connection with your menstrual blood?

❭ How can you create a loving, curious, compassionate, non-judgmental container for yourself to nurture any resistances that may arise?

❭ Have there been phases of dark winter in your life? What did you learn from the hibernation process?

❭ What was your mother's and grandmother's relationship to their menstrual cycle, and how has this impacted your relationship with your womb?

Moon Blood Ritual

A beautiful way to immerse yourself in your inner wisdom is by holding a moon ritual each month at the closing of your moon time. Here are some guided suggestions for offering your moon blood back to Mother Earth in a Moon Planting Ritual, *Siembra de Luna*. You can gather friends or embark on a solo journey if you feel called. Throughout your menstrual cycle, you can collect as much menstrual blood as you can into an airtight glass jar (if you use a menstrual cup, this will be easy; pour the blood into the jar each time you remove your cup). You will have a jar full of vibrant menstrual blood at the end of your cycle.

Now it's time to pack up your moon ritual bag. You may want to bring candles, a lighter, paper or a notebook, your moon blood journal, incense, crystals, musical instruments, oracle decks—anything that feels sacred to you. Perhaps you can choose at least one object to invoke each of the four elements. Choose a spot in nature where you can be calm and uninterrupted (this can look like a small garden, a large forest, a favorite tree, an ocean shoreline, or a rocky mountain) and give yourself plenty of time to hold space for whatever would like to emerge. As you walk to your desired location, pay attention to how Pachamama welcomes you into her home and allows you to receive her guidance. Take time as you notice the color schemes and textures of this territory, and observe the sounds of the wind, the chirps of the birds, and the blossoming of the flowers.

Listen to your intuition, and you will know where to stop. When a space welcomes you, root yourself and build your moon blood altar. You can create an altar gathering nature treasures like sticks, flowers, leaves, and rocks by asking for permission and picking sparingly. Design your altar in a way that feels right for you, and when it is ready, light a candle and sit by the altar.

Allow your inner wisdom to guide you, genuinely trusting in yourself and this process. You may feel called to write, draw, sing, dance, ask for blessings, dive into sobs, or jump for joy. Hold yourself in a compassionate, judgment-free container of curiosity and see what would like to emerge. You may want to use this time to set intentions for your next moon cycle, like planting little seeds to harvest in a future cycle. You may also reflect on last month's seeds of intentions, celebrate transformations, and create space for any restructuring that may want to surface.

Whenever you are ready, you can take your jar of moon blood and intuitively pour it over your altar, offering it in divine connection to Mother Earth. Envision the Earth receiving all that no longer serves you and transmuting this energy into the clearest visions of your most empowered self.

Observe the feelings that arise as you nourish the Earth with such an intimate part of your inner world. You may want to dip your fingers into the blood before or after releasing it to the altar and listen to its messages.

By praying with your moon blood, you are in direct connection with the prayers of the Earth. As you offer your blood back to the Mother, she soaks up your prayers and sends them deep into the dark roots below the surface. From there, they can begin to rise to the creator through the infinitely extending branches and limbs reaching toward the sky. Be careful what you pray for, trusting that your prayers are already being answered. Depending on where you have chosen to build your altar, you may want to visit this space frequently throughout your cycle to remain grounded in your prayers as you spiral through your cycle.

Stories

Blood At Your Front Door

Nine months into my travels, I arrived at a small town where the Colombian Andes meet the Amazon. As the day began, the sky was covered in thick, gray, drizzly clouds. The Mother was grieving with me. I felt my moon coming. I noticed my increased sensitivity toward masculine energies and how I felt impacted by living in a dark house with only men. I walked down into town and made aimless rounds, feeling alone, sad, and lost. I couldn't understand why being by myself felt so empty at this moment.

At times, my solo journey through South America felt liberating, expansive, and full of infinite magic. I had just moved from the sacred Ecuadorian mountains, where I lived near a crystalline river, in a community with my dearly loved brothers and sisters. We held ceremonies, played with

children, danced, and made music. We bathed naked in the
river, learned from plant medicines, and performed live music
together in town. We ate an abundance of delicious tropical
fruits and vegetables and always cooked delicious meals
together. My heart felt so full, and I noticed myself becoming
attached to this experience, unable to accept or understand
why such a beautifully healing and abundant cycle must
come to a close. Weeks before I knew it would end (because
everyone had plans to carry on their journey to other parts
of the Earth, and my Ecuadorian visa was expiring), I began
to feel fear and witnessed the little girl within me wishing for
a miracle fairy tale where we could all stay in those sacred
mountains and live together forever happily ever after.

At times, I felt the weight of this solo journey as a heavy
burden, feeling the grief of displacement and loneliness
wearing on me. As I grieved the end of the beautiful chapter
in the sacred Ecuadorian Andes and missed my friends with
a painful longing in my heart, I decided to take a hike down
to a new unexplored river for some flowing water medicine.
I walked for what seemed like hours. Finally, after a long
journey into the valley, I arrived at a little piece of wood with
an arrow that said RIO (river). The arrow pointed toward a
steep, slippery downhill trail through a coffee plantation. It
seemed impossible to go down that path, but I gave it a shot.
I slipped onto my butt numerous times. I was only wearing
a dress and sandals and felt I could not continue this way.
So I turned around, returned to that little wooden sign, and
looked around. I took in the sound of the river below, so close
yet so far. I observed the large tropical mountains all around
me. I saw a waterfall in the distance. And I felt so small in the
middle of this immense coffee plantation.

Suddenly, I began wailing. I cried hard and yelled,
"Great Spirit, I do not understand! I trust the divine plan,
but I don't understand why I am here now! Give me some

guidance, please!" I cried, cried, and cried. Finally, I decided to continue walking and begin my return up the mountain. And then it started to rain hard. I took refuge from the storm under a giant orange tree. I picked an orange, and as I peeled and ate her flesh, I felt her juices dribbling down my chin and dripping toward my elbow.

I took out my small jade pipe, and I decided to consult Mother Ganja. "Mother, I do not understand why I feel so empty right now if I have received so much love throughout my life, and in the center of my being, I know that there is an infinite fountain of love. How can I access this love stored in my being so that I can fill myself up in these moments of solitude? With this medicine, I release the past and my worries about the future and return to the beauty of this present moment, the only moment that exists. I am grateful to be here now." I inhaled so much nourishment that I had received from many loved ones and exhaled, releasing attachment. This love stays with me, and the rest goes with the wind. I cannot continue to hug something so tightly that no longer exists. I inhaled an abundance of love deep within my being, spiraling outward in expansion and returning to my center. I exhaled peace, and I reminded myself that all is well.

The rain paused a bit, and I decided to continue. I began walking uphill, and eventually, I realized I had taken a wrong turn and was lost deep in a coffee plantation. It began to pour again, so I removed my glasses, which were covered in raindrops. I continued walking up, trusting that there must be an exit, maybe a new path from above. I walked, slipped, got up, and fell again. I walked until I arrived at a giant stone wall towering over me, the end of the path.

At that point, I realized this wasn't the right way and that I had also lost my glasses. I had no idea where on this giant plantation they could be. It seemed symbolic that I had displaced the lenses through which I saw my world. Perhaps I was being asked to see things from a new perspective. I did not expect to find them, yet I did not give up my hope that they could reappear. I couldn't see well, it was raining, and I couldn't even remember which path I had taken. I walked down, looking carefully at the alive, green jungle floor, searching for my glasses, with no luck.

And then, a long while later, I saw them on the ground! This was enough to fill my being with gratitude.

I continued walking down, down, down to the main path. As I took the main trail up, I crossed my arms, hugging myself, soothing and mothering myself. Tears streamed down my face again, but they felt like new and different tears. I no longer felt so alone. I no longer felt that I was the Aviva who allowed herself to be guided by her fears. This Aviva is, of course, a part of me, and I am also accompanied by Aviva who is Mother and Warrior. She hugged me and said, "I am here. I know that you are moving through a challenging moment. You have the right to feel sad and alone. But I am always here with you. We are a team. You are not alone." With that, I continued walking another two hours uphill until I returned home.

When I walked into the house, no one even turned to greet me. One guy did ask me how it went for me at the river, and I started to share something with him, but he didn't listen or respond. I walked toward my room and lay down exhausted on the floor of my patio. There was not a single cloud in the sky. The blue heavens opened up, and the sun shone through.

The next day, I woke up to receive my moon blood. My blood, a deeper understanding of the premenstrual storm that had taken me on such a turbulent ride, had finally arrived to bring some calm and rest. I spent the morning at home and walked down into town wearing nothing more than a long floral dress and carrying some coins in my hand to buy fruit.

Then, unexpectedly, I crossed paths with a beautiful man I had met a few days earlier. He was on his motorcycle, and when he saw me, he pulled over and asked if I wanted to hop on and accompany him to his house up in the mountains. I felt resistance because I was with my moon and didn't feel prepared for a grand adventure. Yet inevitably, I decided to say yes, let's do it.

We arrived at his home, and it began to get dark, so we built a big sacred bonfire. Since it was getting late, a part of me felt nervous about being alone in the middle of the mountain with a man I barely knew. I felt fear and simultaneous surrender. Nevertheless, we connected in an easeful way, creating music, laughing, and talking about sacred plant medicines we had sat with and how they supported our path of healing and love. As it got later, we placed a big cushion with many blankets and pillows next to the fire, and we lay there watching the stars. We cuddled into each other, and I felt warmth in my heart. While I felt attraction toward him, I felt no desire to engage sexually. First, because I was in my process with my moon time. Second, I felt sure that the next time I invited anyone's sexual energy into my womb space, we would be bathed in a light of deep trust and pure intentions.

This night, sexual energies moved in the dark. Although some part of him was interested in my entire being, I noted how easily he allowed himself to be guided plainly by his sexual desires and that he saw in me a way to meet his sexual impulses, regardless of what I wanted. I expressed that I did not want to move sexual energy, and while I felt that he heard me, he did not accept what I said. Many times throughout the night, he tried to touch my body sexually, and I kept repeating my no. He acted as if he touched me in the right way, he could seduce me, and I would want to have sex with him, completely ignoring that I had expressed no interest in engaging sexually.

I felt so turned off that he could not respect my "no." His inability to respect my boundaries affirmed my lack of desire to share any sexual energy with him. Although I still had the urge to sleep next to each other under the stars and cuddle, I did not want to have sex. He repetitively asked me if I would take out my menstrual cup so we could have sex, and I soon shifted from feeling playfully dismissive to frustrated.

My wise, bleeding body accompanied me all night. And in the morning, my blood had a lot to say. I felt my uterus and vaginal canal had contracted in defense mode. So when I went to remove my cup, I felt it buried deep inside me. I stood right at the house's entrance because directly next to the door was a hose I could use to rinse out my cup. I began to pull on the cup with force, and suddenly, the whole cup exploded inside me, and all the blood spilled everywhere.

Red blood dripping on the ground, red blood dripping on my legs, red blood dripping on my dress. I went quickly to turn on the hose, but no water came out! Within a few seconds, the dog came and began to lick the puddle of blood on the floor. Panicked, I tried to pick up the blood with my hands and smeared it more. I attempted to wash my hands in the sink inside the house (leaving a little trail of blood drops), but no water came through there either.

And in the midst of it all, the man came back and found me standing naked, my blood-covered dress thrown at the front door of his house, and my menstrual cup in hand, dripping blood everywhere. I explained what had happened, and he went to open the water tanks, explaining that he had shut off the water through the night. He received me with a lot of compassion. He gave me a towel and turned on the shower for me. He had switched from aggressively wanting something from me to being of service to me. As I showered, I chuckled at this scene as if my blood showed him and me my true power. I had never experienced my menstrual cup exploding in that kind of way. Still, perhaps that blood was exploding and creating this mess on my behalf, for all those times I internalized men surpassing my sexual limits. I had been socialized to swallow my discomfort and stay quiet to avoid making a scene. But this time, the power of my blood spoke, yelled, cried, and celebrated for me.

Plan B: My First Siembra de Luna

I have gone through just two moon cycles since taking out my IUD. I feel my body's beauty reentering into a sacred cyclical rhythm. I am gaining a deeper understanding of the ebbs and flows of my hormonal waves. I see myself each day as a cyclically-empowered woman.

After leaving Colombia, I traveled south to a small rural indigenous town in the northern part of the Ecuadorian Andes. The town center is known for holding South America's largest artisanal market, and the surrounding nature is home to endless green hills, flowing rivers, and sacred waterfalls.

As my bus pulled into the outskirts of the town, I decided to get off because I saw a man dressed as a clown juggling at the traffic light. Whenever I saw musicians, circus performers, and artisans on the street, I assumed they were artist backpackers, *mochileros*, like me, and may know of a nice communal non-tourist place to stay. So I got out and began speaking to him, and he told me he was staying at a humble traveler's hostel by the river. He had been juggling for a few hours, and his pockets were heavy with coins, so he offered to walk with me toward the hostel. When we arrived, there were only a few other men and no women, making me uneasy. But I appreciated that I could have a private room and felt extremely held by the beauty of the surrounding nature. So I decided to stay.

As I tell this story, I am working hard on forgiving myself, feeling self-judgment arise about the endless series of self-harming decisions I began to make, acting in risky ways with men, with my heart, sexual energy, and body temple.

The next day, I connected with a random guy from the hostel. I didn't feel physically or sexually attracted to him, but I enjoyed the company and conversation. I am not sure what changed so quickly, but somehow, we ended up having sex just hours after we had met, and we didn't use a condom. After that experience, I felt a lot of shame and did not want to have sex with him again or relate to him romantically.

Later that night, all the men were drunk when I came home to the hostel. He came to me and attempted to touch my body in a highly sexual way, and I felt uncomfortable and defensive. I was the only woman staying at the hostel, and I felt unsafe around these drunk, sexualized men. So I went to my room and tried to sleep over the sound of yelling and loud music.

Suddenly, this man burst open my room door and tried to enter my bed. I felt startled but confidently asked him to leave and locked the door behind him. The following day, unsure of how and where to take my next steps, clearly needing space from this hostel, I packed a small bag and prepared to go into town for the rest of the day.

In town, I sang songs with my ukulele at the restaurants surrounding the market during lunch hour. I made money by sharing my music and bought incredible jewelry and hand-woven clothing. Then, I met an artisan man who I began speaking to and spending some time with.

As I write and feel disgust for myself, I also call in compassion for myself and these men, knowing that underlying all of the toxicity that arose, there was simply a need for connection, belonging, intimacy, and trust. So, as the conversation went on with this man, he offered to give me a free hair wrap, and then, as it got dark, he asked if I wanted to come over for dinner. While I didn't really know or fully trust him, his energy was calm, and I was in no rush to return to my threatening hostel, so I said yes. We ended up cooking a meal back at his home, and then he offered that I spend the night. I felt hesitation, knowing that I had just had sex with a man hours after meeting him, and then I felt deep guilt and shame toward myself. However, I also felt I could spend the night without having sex, so I said yes.

That night, we simply slept next to each other, and in the morning, I felt celebratory that there hadn't been any surpassing of my sexual boundaries.

Then, within minutes of waking, we began having sex.

I must have been extremely lonely because I had never felt attracted to or inspired by this man. Whether moving sexual energy or not, I felt disconnected, disgusted, and ashamed throughout our time together. Still, I thought it was a good idea to accept his offer to take all my things out of the nearby hostel and move in with him. We spent a bizarre week together, where he showed me his possessiveness, jealousy, manipulation, anxiety, and depression.

I felt so lost in myself. Somehow, I began to tell myself the story that this was okay for me.

What part of me felt so unworthy that I was willing to tolerate this toxic relationship?

All the while, we were having sex without a condom. He always managed to pull out before ejaculating, but one night, he came inside me. Instantly, I pushed him off me, and I felt stunned, speechless, and paralyzed for a few minutes. Then I started sobbing. This finally was the breaking point for me. What was I doing having unprotected sex with this man I felt deep disgust toward?

It finally clicked that we were engaging in an act that could create life within me. I felt such deep fear, anger, and sadness. I had never had any man ejaculate inside of me without protective birth control. I felt this image of myself as an empowered cyclical medicine woman crash down in front of me, and I melted into a helpless puddle on the Earth.

I was only beginning to explore the rhythm of my cycle and hadn't experienced enough cycles to know with certainty when my fertile window was. I went straight to my moon chart and noted that I was on day 11, which could have been a fertile day. I was sure that I would absolutely not risk the option of becoming pregnant with this man's child and came up with the solution of taking Plan B. This felt like a horrible option, knowing the hormonal imbalances that would impact my body, which was just beginning to return to its normal rhythm. I also felt this was an emergency since I had never taken Plan B and never planned to take it again.

That night, I still slept in his bed and felt some forgiveness about the whole thing. This would have been an excellent opportunity to pack up everything the next morning and move on with my journey, but instead, together, we woke up early and went straight into town to buy a Plan B pill at a pharmacy. He seemed hesitant that I take this emergency contraceptive pill and even encouraged me not to take it, saying he would support me if I became pregnant with his child. This was strange. We met one week ago, and he was open to having a child with me. He was over ten years older than me and lived a lonely life. It was almost as if he wished I would have his child, so I couldn't leave him. Ultimately, he said the choice was mine. So we awkwardly went to a pharmacy together to ask for the pill and had to explain to the blushing nurse that we had unprotected sex, and he came inside of me, and I was potentially in my fertile window.

I am grateful that he was willing to accompany me throughout the process, and I recognize how vulnerable this whole experience was for me and why I may have felt a need for company. But still, I question where the bold, courageous, and self-trusting part of me was hiding. What I wish my most empowered self had done in that moment was say goodbye and move on, but we decided to spend the rest of the day together until the afternoon when we ran into a friend I knew at the market. He was a musician I had just met, so I didn't know him too well, but I appreciated our mutual love for Andean music, and when he asked if I wanted to come over to make some music, I excitedly responded yes.

I felt I was beginning to emerge from this dark hole of creepy men I had dug myself into. He invited me to his hostel, the same hostel I had stayed at previously. I didn't feel too excited about going back there, but at this point, I needed an uplifting creative connection to sink back into ease and playfulness within myself.

Unfortunately, when I told the Plan B guy that I would make music with a friend, he became verbally abusive and acted like I was his property and that he could control and decide what I could or could not do. That attitude freaked me out and was exactly the push I needed to get my stuff and leave his home for good. But it was already super late and dark, and I felt too scared to return to his house alone. So I decided to see my musician friend and risk whatever the repercussions may be the following day.

When I arrived at the hostel, the musician asked me if I wanted to take a walk, to which I shared a total yes, feeling no need to spend time at that hostel. I expressed to this new friend the strange and somewhat dangerous situation I was currently in, and as soon as it was morning, I knew that I would need to go back to Plan B's house, quickly pack up my things, and get far away from this town. This friend seemed supportive as he listened and hugged me.

We continued walking into a dark forest and sat on a big rock. Then he leaned over, tried to kiss me, and touched my breasts with this wild, uncontrolled machista sexual energy. I told him clearly and calmly that I had no desire to engage in sexual activity with him, and immediately, I could tell he wasn't listening. He continued to touch me in sexual ways, and I kept saying no. I felt that I was trapping myself into some cruel, nonconsensual game where I would say no, he would completely disregard my boundaries, and I would still stay.

It is challenging to avoid telling this story from a victim-blaming perspective since, as I write, I feel myself adamantly encouraging myself to get up and go! What could have been more empowering than honoring my clear no and moving toward a clear yes in that moment? I know I felt deep fear and vulnerability paralyzing me and creating obstacles to acting from an empowered place. But I wonder what wounded part of me that needed love continued to stay time after time with that man after my sexual boundaries were continuously being violated.

From this place of fear, I somehow decided to spend the night with this guy. (Since it was already the middle of the night, I told myself the false story that there was "nowhere else to go.") Now I know that there is always somewhere else to go that does not involve sleeping in the same bed as a man who has repetitively disrespected my boundaries.

Throughout the night, he continuously stuck his hand up my shirt and down my pants, and I kept having to push him away until finally, morning came, and I felt that the rising sun could accompany this next part of my journey.

Of course, before I left, he kept asking if we could have sex, and I couldn't understand how he could remain so fixated on his sexual needs without considering the endless NO!s I had already given him. So I marched out of there, straight into Plan B's house, and I felt I was in a telenovela scene. I began quickly packing my things as he cried on the floor and begged me to stay. He apologized for many things; the more he cried, the quicker I packed. Finally, he asked if he could come wherever I went, and I said no. I tried to thank him for all I had learned from this experience and wish him well on his journey, but he wasn't accepting that I was leaving and demanded that I stay.

I felt dizzy as I packed, almost as if observing this scene from above. As I somehow managed to pull everything together and say goodbye, I had never walked so quickly to the bus stop without looking back. Right before waiting at the bus stop, I went to pee around the corner, and when I got to the stop, he was already there waiting for me. He had run there insisting on coming with me, and I kept asking him firmly to leave me alone. Finally, a bus pulled up, and I sprinted onto the bus, praying that he wouldn't follow me. As the bus pulled away, I felt my accelerated heart, my nervous system in complete survival mode, and I slowly began to take deeper exhales, telling myself that I was safe. I cried so loudly on the bus, feeling the deep pain of this whole thunderstorm. While many people on the bus looked back at me in curiosity and confusion, no one came to check in with the emotionally distressed gringa in the back.

Eventually, the man who collects the bus fares came over to sobbing me and cold-heartedly asked me to pay. I went to reach for my wallet, and I found it empty as soon as I opened it. Plan B man must have stolen the money from my wallet as I was packing up to trap me and make it impossible for me to leave because it was full of cash this morning. This made me cry more, and the busman stood waiting for me to pay him. Luckily, the fare wasn't too expensive, and I remembered I had a few spare coins left in my ukulele case. With that, I was able to pay the fare and continue my process of sobbing and self-soothing.

When the bus finally arrived at the Quito bus terminal, I knew that I was only a short taxi ride away from the safe home of my Ecuadorian host mother. Yet, I didn't have the cash to pay for the taxi. So, when I got off the bus, I threw all my things onto the floor and cuddled myself into a fetal position while I cried.

There were simple action steps I could have taken at the time, like calling my host mom and asking for support or finding an ATM and retrieving cash. But my brain felt so shocked from being in survival mode that I couldn't think clearly, and the only thing I could do was cry on the floor of the bus terminal.

Eventually, this badass butch lesbian approached me and firmly asked me what was happening. Through sobs, I briefly explained that I was coming out of a dark portal with toxic men and that I needed to get to my host mom's house nearby but had no money for the taxi. She told me she was heading in that direction and would take the bus. She grabbed one of my bags and then urged me to follow her. So I picked myself up while still whimpering and followed her as she paid for two bus tickets and made way for me to continue her lead. Once on the bus, she shared some of the traumatic experiences she had lived with men and explained why she never trusted any men. She shared that she and her female partner always kept their guard around men and even encouraged me not to trust any man. This was her story, so I appreciated her support and took her suggestions with a grain of salt. Eventually, my stop came, and I got off to walk home. I was visiting my Ecuadorian family, whom I had lived with for six months, about a year and a half ago. Arriving there meant a clean, safe, private space where I could be nourished, slow down, and show up just as I was. Just a short walk home, and I could completely let my guard down.

This was a challenging chapter for me. Unfortunately, it did not neatly resolve as quickly or as easily as I would have wished in the coming weeks. After resting and recharging for a few days, I traveled to a small beach town. I had another entangling sexual interaction with a man with whom I felt disgusted. He was a fire-breather and permanently reeked of gasoline. While we had sex, I inevitably developed a vaginal fungal infection, my womb's way of warning me to slow down and be mindful of who I was inviting into my body. I kept anxiously counting down the days until my body bled. I prayed that Mother Earth would bring me my moon cycle, and in turn, I promised to offer my blood back to her. Although I had taken Plan B, I wouldn't feel confident that I had avoided pregnancy until my menstruation came.

One day, I felt increasingly irritable, and my breasts began feeling super tender. Later that night, I felt my belly bloat and my uterus cramping. I was sure I would start my moon cycle the next day, and sure enough, upon waking, I began bleeding. I had never felt such deep relief, gratitude, and celebration to allow my body to cleanse itself and release the pain I had stored up throughout my last cycle. I knew some of it was my wounding, but I also carried the weight of four men's burdens with whom I had shared sexual interactions the previous month.

As I bled into my menstrual cup, I gathered my moon blood in a glass jar. I packed a bag for my first-ever moon blood ritual a few days later. I walked away from the ocean toward a small area with big coastal trees, and along the way, I picked up some feathers and shells that I would offer to Mother Earth along with my blood.

I set up an altar and sang many songs my Colombian witchy sisters had passed on to me. I set an intention to bury, along with my blood, my sense of unworthiness, self-hatred, shame, and guilt, and asked La Pachamama to allow me to transform all of this pain into more profound love for myself and others. I prayed that with the burial of this moon, I could receive guidance to continue walking my soul's true path so that I may serve the Great Spirit. I watched parts of myself ascend in the sacred smoke of the palo santo. I cried, I celebrated, and when I felt a sense of completion, I walked away with gratitude.

As I emerged from this ceremony, I felt relief, lightness, and self-trust. I walked back toward the ocean with a more profound sense of self-confidence that I could use the blood within my body to create magic and bridge the spiritual and material worlds.

A few minutes into my walk, I directly crossed paths with the Plan B man! I felt shocked and in disbelief that after holding so much space for him in the ceremony and praying for forgiveness and compassion, he appeared in front of me minutes later. Interestingly, I felt I was no longer the woman I was a few weeks ago. Especially after this powerful moon blood ritual, I did not feel fear upon seeing him. Instead, I walked past him without acknowledging him, having no desire to interact. At that moment, I felt supercharged and electric, as if the Great Spirit had given me a big hug of protection and reminded me, "There is nothing to be afraid of, my child. I will guide you if you are willing to listen." The message was evident. Shortly after, I left that beach town and continued on a long journey toward Vilcabamba, a small mountain town in the Southern Ecuadorian Andes.

Menstruation is Grief

Winter 2020 is turning into Spring, and I just got my long-awaited period after days of feeling late. I imagined that I could have gotten pregnant. Even though we hadn't had penetrative sex, my partner and I had penis and vagina contact post-ejaculation on the day I was ovulating. I spoke about my deep desire to become a mother with the vibrant orgasmic glow of post-sexy time creation energy. Even though the circumstance of becoming pregnant at this moment seemed ridiculous and improbable, it felt profoundly moving and emotional for me. Had the Great Spirit heard my prayers in that powerful post-sex portal? I meant I wanted to be a mother... eventually... not right now! Still, I felt an activation of total readiness and openness to receiving this potential life. I also felt fear and doubt, but this strong maternal instinct spoke louder than any other voice, making me feel held and confident that I was ready to become a mother. I imagined this beautiful little child being my adventure buddy, playing the ukulele, dancing with me, running naked in the garden, swimming in the cold river, and juggling hula hoops.

When my moon blood came, I wept. And I understood how menstruation is grief. This blood is my body grieving not being a mother. My body had prepared this delicious fertile lining for life, for a beating heart to birth within me so I could nurture it with infinite compassionate love. And then, when my egg was not fertilized, my body went into destruction mode, tearing down the lining. So when this blood finally poured through me, I knew that this was the purest offering I could return to Mother Earth. My menstrual blood carried my fertile life force creation energy straight from my womb heart center back to the Great Mother of all life on Earth.

This experience led me to a deep reconnection with the magic of my blood. I wanted to smear it on my body, cover cave walls, paint canvases, build an altar, and pour it back into the Earth with so much awareness of how powerful this intentional fluid is. I felt such a deep appreciation of the magic of my cyclical body and a whisper of mourning if my period were ever to leave me for a while.

This moon shifted the way I see myself and the things I am capable of nurturing right now in this present moment. I felt so supported imagining writing to all these beautiful humans I hold with deep love in my heart that I was going to have a baby. The vision was strikingly clear and full of prayer and magic. I witnessed myself surrounded by sacred mountains, plant medicines, natural birth doulas, and many other wild children running naked through crystalline waters.

I feel truly grateful and humbled to have had the tools to experience this late period as sensations in my body and gain a new awareness about my needs and desires, like gaining a true North without attaching to the form and structure. There were little details that were fun and warming to imagine. Still, primarily, my response to the possibility of being pregnant (and having the child) demonstrated to me how trusting I feel of my inner strength, how willing and ready I am to nurture another human with love, and how much work there is still for me to do in healing my relationship to men. I desire that in whatever form he may come, I may deeply trust the father as an equally wise, loving partner in creating life. I also see how much of my healing I would love to integrate before passing a life through my body, and I surrender to the mystery as it unfolds.

I have included the lyrics to a song I wrote as a way to process bleeding as grief:

All of My Phases

My blood's coming down with grief today
I am releasing, creating space
Shedding, letting go of all that no longer serves me
Rebirthing into all that I was ever meant to be
I am transforming the pain and the shame
Riding the waves of intensity with grace
As I embrace
All of my phases
As I make love
To all of these changes
I am here singing the song
And I am dancing the dance
With the ancient ones
Remembering the wisdom we've known all along
Spilling my waters back toward the mother
May you transmute my tears and my blood
May you hold me in your compassionate arms
May you guide me as I swim through your darkness

On Your Shoreline

On January 5, 2022, at 7:30 p.m. in Puerto Viejo, Costa Rica, I went to the beach alone. I plopped my stuff down near a well-lit restaurant, yet still, I was in the darkness. So I decided to take my clothes off and play naked in the ocean. This was the Caribbean, so the water was warm, and bioluminescent lights danced on the shoreline. I sent all my prayers through the great Mother Ocean, *Madre Mar*, *Yemanja*. I felt her mystical magic in the waves crashing in the dark. I heard her song in such a unique way, distinct from her daytime lullabies. I harmonized with the crash of the waves and felt held and safe by her majestic expanse.

I returned to get my clothes, shaking my body to dry off a little. Then, suddenly, I felt a man come up behind me and say, *"Mira a ese cuerpo...* Look at that body." He shined a cell phone light on me, scanning me up and down as if I were some barcode. I started to say to him firmly and loudly, *"Véte, déjame en paz...* Go away, leave me alone," to which he responded violently, *"Cállate, no hagas mucho ruido...* Shut up, don't make a lot of noise." So then I crouched down to cover my exposed naked body, and he came to my front, shined a light right between my legs, and said, *"Déjame ver esa conchita...* Let me see your little pussy." And then I started screaming with so much vehement force that I could only have imagined carrying all this power within.

My soul released a cry of emergency survival mode. My body immediately responded to protect myself. As I began screaming, he got up and appeared as if he were going to run away, but then he came in from behind me and started painfully jabbing his fingers into my vagina. I quickly moved my body and screamed, *"Ayudaaaa...* Heeeelp," thousands of decibels louder than before. Then he sprinted away while simultaneously a group of people from the restaurant began walking toward me and asking from a distance, *"Todo bien?...* Is everything okay?"

My body began trembling uncontrollably, and I lost my breath, slipping into hyperventilation. I felt my nervous system's code red alarm buzzing with every mechanism possible to signal, emergency, emergency, emergency—we are not safe!!! Through shaking limbs and sobs, I tried to get dressed and communicate to the people who had approached me that I had just been assaulted. As I wept, continued screaming, and embarked on the impossible task of catching my breath while putting my clothes on, I asked if they could accompany me back to my bike. Once I got on the bike, I was only five minutes away from home. I peddled so quickly that it felt like one minute. At the gate of my neighborhood, a neighbor was outside, about to hop on her bike in the opposite direction. Yet, seeing me in my condition and hearing my wails and hyperventilation coming up the road, she accompanied me through the gate, soothingly touching my back and grabbing my bike. We walked over to my next-door neighbor's house, and together, these two women embraced me, held me, and repeated, "You are safe here." They took me onto their porch, brought me water and tea, and gave me space to find my breath and share my story. After time had passed and I felt okay to sleep, I thanked them for being my angels and then went to my bedroom.

There, I began to replay the scenario and became consumed by fear and grief in that dark room. A new wave of panic and trauma washed over me. Again, I couldn't stop crying, and my normal breath escaped me. My other neighbor knocked on the door and offered me some company. I received it with deep gratitude and cuddled into her as I wept. I repeated the story of what had happened, feeling that there would be many instances where I recounted this story in the next several days. She offered to spend the night with me so that I may feel safe and held.

The next morning, I awoke to all kinds of emotions and questions. One major thing to celebrate is that I have my voice. I have been assaulted many times before and often felt so shocked and paralyzed that I had found it nearly impossible to use my voice. My body had relied on a defense mechanism of shutting down and checking out. In the past, when the perpetrators had told me to be silent, I had feared speaking out, afraid that they might lash out at me with more violence. Yet, I didn't even have to think about screaming last night. My voice was so open that I instantly unlocked it to save myself. The fear inflicted upon me to remain silent during the assault had often remained in my body far after the assault. During one rape years ago in Ecuador, he kept covering my mouth to be silent, so I listened and remained silent for months. When he finished raping me, and I came home to find my host mom and sister having tea at the table, I joined them and acted like nothing unusual had happened. I don't even remember shedding a single tear.

This familiar trauma has reappeared for me to heal this recurring wound completely. Maybe I needed this experience in the present moment to process this trauma in a fully embodied way, share my story, scream, ask for help, and take up the space that I never claimed after so many years of being silenced. I have experienced minor consent violations in the last few years, but nothing too violent or traumatizing. I felt proud to cultivate a deep sense of safety and trust within my body. As if I were an addict who had been sober for a few years, I was a survivor who had been a few years free of sexual assault. Living through sexual trauma has led me to the deep healing of my womb space, reconnection to my bleeding body, and pointed me on the path to writing *Moon Blood*, and for all of this, I am grateful. And some part of me also wholeheartedly thought that I had somehow "ascended" this trauma. I felt that I had done enough work to sit with, heal, love, and transform these wounded parts of myself, and I was no longer buzzing from the same hurt place that would energetically attract others with similar traumas.

I feel genuine gratitude for every single moment of this life that I have lived and everything that has been a teacher to me. Pain, suffering, and trauma are incredible teachers. And I pray to the Great Spirit to also invite in an abundance of joy, beauty, juicy ecstatic pleasure, playfulness, connection, and synchronous magic as my teachers. What is it that my karmic soul is here to learn as I pass through this turn of the spiral again? How can I reap the lessons without personalizing this so much about "my journey"? I know that it is vital for me to reflect and heal and hold space for what needs to arise in my process. And I also understand that this is way bigger than "me." It's not even about "me."

This is a collective wound, and scenarios like this and worse are playing out on Earth every day. (Later, I found out that this very night at this same beach, just a few minutes after me, two gringa women were kidnapped off the beach and raped). I know that someone who re-enacts violence toward another can only act this way because they have been violated. They, too, carry wounds, and since they haven't had the support to heal and integrate them, they seek to project this pain and inflict their suffering on others. But just because someone carries pain inside, they cannot make it magically disappear by giving it to someone else. Our pain is one, as is our collective healing process. So, as much as I am traumatized by the events that occurred last night, I know I have the tools to hold myself and seek support from my community.

Yet, I feel deep compassion and sorrow for the perpetrators of violence. I know some feel guilt and shame for their behavior, but it's risky to feel those feelings because they would open up an infinite portal of grief they may not be willing to face, especially alone. I understand the coping mechanism of numbness that both the perpetrator and the survivor use to subside the big and uncomfortable emotions.

So, how can we continue to heal together? How can we implement compassionate, loving, restorative justice therapies in which those with deep trauma aren't labeled as "criminals," "crazy," or "bad people" but instead recognized as full humans needing to be seen and loved?

We cannot heal alone when we are all sharing the same Earth, the same water, and the same air.

Our processes are all intertwined.

May we live in a world where it is safe to occupy our bodies.

May we live in a world where being naked is not inherently sexual.

May we live in a world where all beings are free of suffering.

May we live in a world deeply embedded in the wisdom of compassion so that we may remember that everything we create in our external reality expresses our inner worlds and vice versa.

May we all know true inner peace and liberation.

I hold in my heart that every step of the way supports my healing journey and the evolution of my soul, and this event is no exception. Maybe I needed to go through an event like this to be reminded why I am so moved to write *Moon Blood*, share my journey, and support others in healing their womb space and rediscovering the beauty within their cyclical being. Maybe this reminds me of how unbelievably strong my voice is and how resilient I am. Perhaps this is a reminder that regardless of how many years or lifetimes go by, I carry the identity of a survivor of assault, and it is part of my calling on this Earth to hold space for these ancestral wounds and allow them to move through me as I ascend in my spiral. Maybe it is a sobering reminder to celebrate my discernment and care for the spaces and people I am opening my vulnerable and trusting self.

As I embark on a new journey to Guatemala, and my body begins to bleed, I acknowledge that every part of my life is a part of me. I am allowed to take up space when I am grieving. I am allowed to take up space in my radiant ovulatory glow. I am allowed to bring my whole self and all of my stories, and I am free to leave them behind and begin anew.

Rebirth

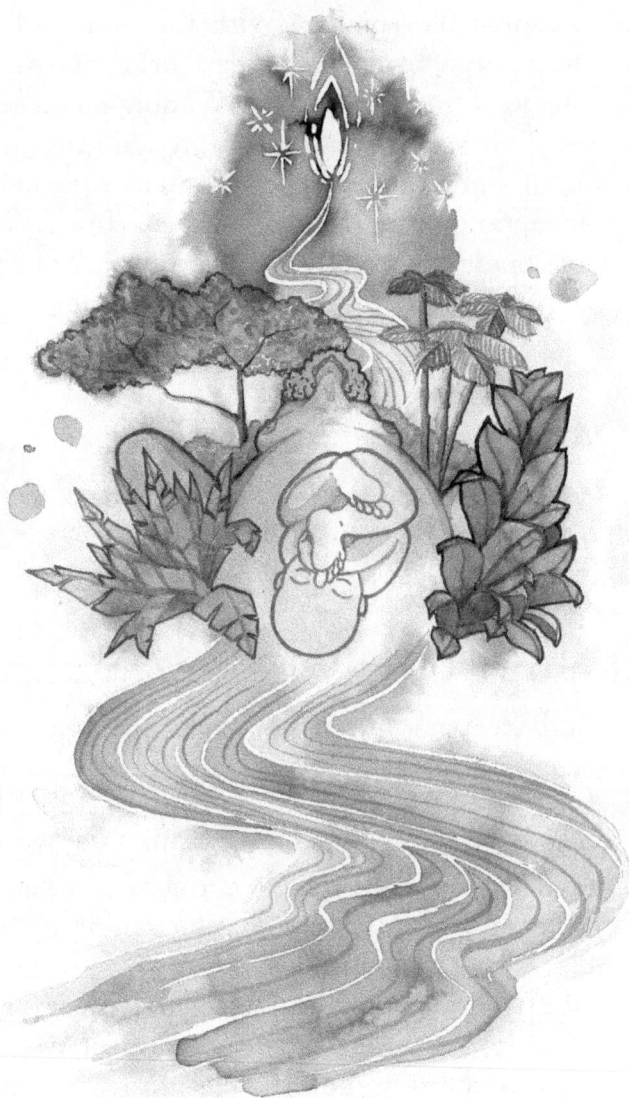

Moon's Energy

With the rising light of the waxing moon (approximately days 7-14 of the moon cycle), vibrant, youthful energy nourishes personal blossoming. With this renewed energy, you begin to emerge from the inner world you have been cocooning inside of throughout your Waning moon and New moon phases. This is a perfect moment to gain the embodied practice of nourishing the seeds you planted in the new moon with aligned action steps. Rejoice and celebrate, knowing that you have made it through the darkest part of the cycle and are now fully emerging into the brightest phases.

Moon Phase: Waxing

The Waxing moon is our transition from the dark New to the bright Full moon. Each night will become slightly more illuminated as we build up to our fullest peak.

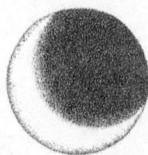

Menstrual Cycle Phase: Pre-Ovulation

In a womb keeper's menstrual cycle, the pre-ovulation/follicular phase begins a few days after menstrual bleeding has ceased. Fluid-filled sacs in your ovaries called follicles pour their energy into maturing an egg that will be released in ovulation. The dominant follicle containing a mature egg increases estrogen within your body, thickening your uterus lining so an egg may implant there.

As a result, you may finally feel fertile energy growing within your body, a genuine desire to connect with others, an increased sexual desire, and the strength and capacity to manifest your intentions.

Cervical Dance

A few days after menstruation has ceased, there may be little to no cervical fluid. This stage is typically referred to as the "dry days." However, days before reaching your fertile peak, your cervix should begin to produce some cervical fluid. All bodies are different, so you must track your cycle to discover your particular flow. Often, your body may transition out of your dry days into slightly fertile cervical fluid. This fluid might be creamy, gluey, sticky, thick, white, or crumbly. Sometimes, the body jumps from dry days to extremely fertile cervical fluid. This fluid might be clear, translucent, sticky, slinky, slimy, or egg whitey. This is a sign that your body is preparing to ovulate. It is also possible that your body never has dry days, jumping straight from menstruation into slightly fertile fluids.

As your cervix moves into a fertile position, its position should be high, soft, and open.

Season: Springtime

Welcome to springtime after a long, cold winter—a beautiful time to smell the fresh wildflowers in bloom and re-emerge from your inward rest. The land has been resting throughout the Winter and is now calling you to prepare her soil to sew the seeds that will bear fruits in the Summer. My name, Aviva, means Spring in Hebrew, and in Spanish means "to bring life to." As a springtime Aquarius, this is one of my favorite parts of the year and of each cycle. This phase reminds me to celebrate that I have made it through the darkest shadows, and after all of my shedding, I am renewed and prepared to be reborn.

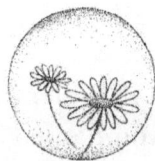

Element: Air

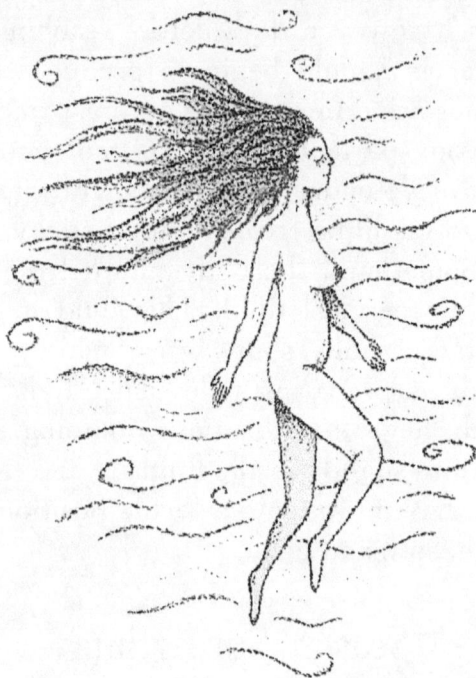

The element for Rebirth is Air. In this phase, you are accompanied by the spirits of birds in flight, free to spread your wings and soar with infinite potential toward manifesting your dreams. Imagine you are the element that stokes the fire. By sharing your breath with a few logs burning low, you have the power to bring embers to a wild flame. The air element also manifests as an active mind in the body. This is a perfect moment to express yourself verbally and use your mind in your favor. Let the air element accompany you, perhaps by keeping feathers near, burning purifying incense, listening to wind instruments, or painting your favorite bird.

Direction: East

This is the portal of the East gate. Here, you are rebirthing with childlike enthusiasm. You may feel inspired and trust that anything is infinitely possible in this direction. This is the direction of the new day, of the rising sun. It is also the direction that all Jews face as they pray, orienting themselves toward the holy city of Jerusalem. You can work on not only cultivating trust at this gate but faith as well. Trust is said to be of the mind, and faith is of the heart.

In the life cycle, this is a newborn child re-emerging into a new life and is represented by yellow. The spirit animals of the East are the Eagle and the Condor. The Eagle carries the medicine from the Northern Hemisphere and embodies a linear, structural, far-sightedness. The Condor carries the medicine from the Southern Hemisphere and symbolizes an intuitive, receptive connection to the Earth. In the prophecy of the Eagle and the Condor, when they fly together, the seemingly opposing systems of North and South will learn to weave together, and a new dawn will shine upon Earth.

Astrological Signs: Air Signs

Gemini: The third Zodiac sign, Gemini, is a cardinal air sign ruled by Mercury, creating space for duality and fluctuations between extremities. The Gemini energy is an excellent portal for mental processing, verbal communication, creative projects, writing, reading, and storytelling. Geminis are "jacks of all trade, masters of none," so you can work with this energy by dipping your toes in diverse creative activities without attaching to anyone.

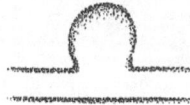

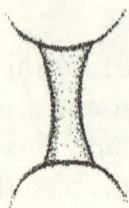

Libra: Libra is the seventh sign of the Zodiac, the second Air sign, and a fixed sign ruled by Venus. Libra's energy is about balance, social order, and harmony in relationships. This is a powerful portal to channel beauty and feminine intuition through your body and your partnerships. Observe how your surroundings mirror your inner world, notice the reflections around you, and connect to the deep well of empathy within.

Aquarius: Aquarius is the eleventh Zodiac sign, the third and final Air sign, a mutable sign ruled by both the structured Saturn and the change-making Uranus. She is the water bearer, fiercely unique, inspired by humanitarian and social causes. Watch for an overactive mind and a tendency to move toward judgment and over-analysis. This powerful portal of freedom creates space to break free from structures that no longer serve us and invite change and innovation with ease.

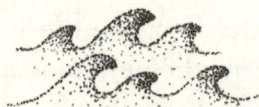

Female Archetype: Wild Child & Maiden

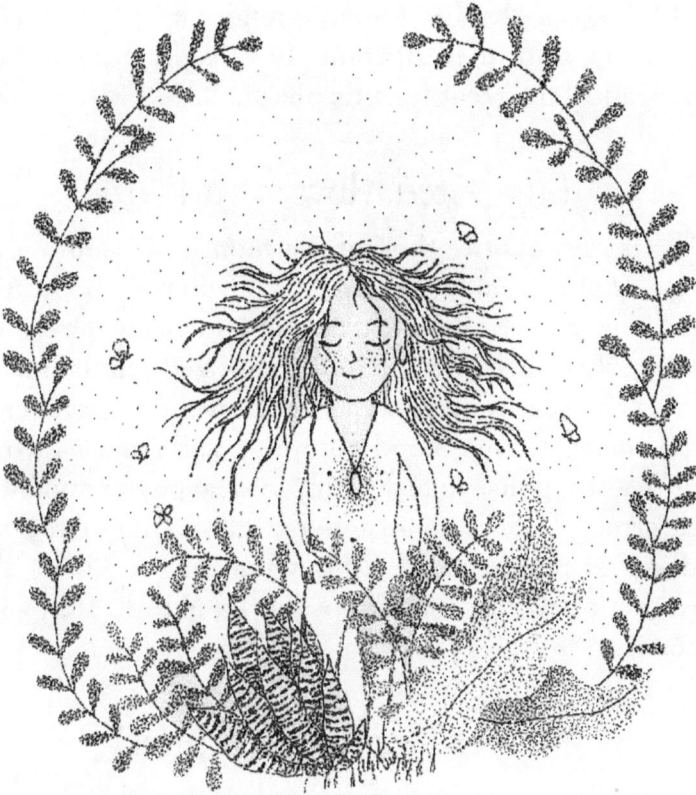

This time resembles the archetype of the virgin or maiden. We are renewed, refreshed, and revitalized since we have just shed and released during our menstruation time. I do not fully resonate with the social concept of the virgin, so I suggest that this archetype is also of a wild child. Envision yourself as a naked little girl splashing near a river, collecting shells, and lathering your body in mud. With this childlike ease, lightness, and curiosity, your most profound power may arise in your following ovulation phase.

Suggested Foods

The follicular phase is about sustaining and nourishing new life, so look for foods containing phytoestrogens, antioxidants, and fiber. Sprouts, flax seeds, pumpkin seeds, and avocados are great for this phase.

Suggested Movement Plan

This is my favorite time of the month to begin an active exercise and movement routine. Typically, my body feels so restored from the premenstrual and menstrual rest that I often eagerly dance into my fully energized self again.

This is a great time to try active movement practices that get your heart racing, blood pumping, and muscles working. This is the best phase to test your physical power and increase muscle strength. So, find an activity that helps you feel strong and discover the pleasure in knowing that you have chosen a movement practice that supports the natural flow of your hormones.

Suggested Herbal Support

For further support in fully embodying the lightness of this phase, I suggest incorporating refreshing and cooling herbs such as Mint, Lemon Grass, Lemon Verbena, Cilantro, and Rosemary. You can also turn to rejuvenating Red Raspberry Leaf high in antioxidants and vitamins, making this a supportive womb herb throughout your entire cycle. You can take these herbs as a tincture, tea, topical salve, or cook with them.

Cyclical Gardening

Since the plant's waters are rising to arrive at the leaves at the full moon, gravity supports the plants to draw up nutrients from the root and send them up to nourish the whole plant. This is a great time to compost the soil so the entire plant can absorb the richness. This is also a great time to graft trees. For example, if you have a tree with strong roots and trunk but have noticed that its branches are not producing much fruit, you can chop a branch of an abundantly-producing fruit tree and graft it onto a chopped branch of the strong tree. When you graft in this phase, the branch's energy will continue to shoot straight up and begin to produce new leaves.

Writing Reflections

- ❭ What practices can you cultivate to connect to the feeling of youthful ease within you?

- ❭ Are there any resistances for you around embodying the archetype of the young maiden?

- ❭ How can you create a loving, curious, compassionate, non-judgmental container for yourself to nurture any resistances that may arise?

- ❭ What memories do you have of playing like a wild child in nature?

- ❭ What fills you with the confidence to create your path?

- ❭ If you could envision the light of a new day dawning all over the Earth, what does this feel like within your body?

Vocal Activation Ritual

In Eastern tradition, the human body is home to seven energy centers, or chakras, starting at the rooted tailbone and flowing up the spine toward the crown of our head. In Sanskrit, the word chakra means "wheel," symbolizing the constant flow of continuously spiraling energy. All these chakras would remain open in a perfectly flowing river, and your energy would gracefully flow from one center to the next. But sometimes life happens, and you may store trauma, painful memories, anger, and resentment within your chakras, which ultimately cause a blockage and prevent the energy from continuously flowing.

Each chakra develops from birth until death, spiraling around every seven years. So, anything that may have impacted the development of a specific chakra at a young age may continue to manifest as a toxic pattern throughout your life until it is recognized and released. Similarly, anything that may have impacted you at seven years old may appear again with striking clarity at 14, 21, etc. While I do not intend to dive deeply into the seven chakra systems, for womb wellness, I want to highlight two specific chakras, the second and the fifth chakra.

The second chakra, associated with the color orange, is the home of your womb space. This is where your sexual organs lie and your creative energy is stored. When this chakra is in balance, you may feel you have access to the infinite well of creativity within you. You may feel inspired, connected to your sensuality, trusting, and expressive. This is the place in your body where human life is created and is a sacred portal to your eternal divinity.

When the second chakra is blocked due to unintegrated womb trauma, you may feel fearful, doubtful, closed off sexually, cut off from your creativity, and shut down in your capacity to feel pleasure. Since your womb is a place of intuition, when this chakra is in balance, you can easily trust your inner wisdom and make empowered decisions about your path. When this chakra is blocked, you may feel confused and lack faith in yourself. The beautiful thing about chakras is that they are a wheel and thrive when free to spin in motion. These energy centers are designed to flow; if you are willing to work with your body, she will support you in clearing blockages.

Sometimes, these blockages ask to be seen, acknowledged, and held in love so they may be released and returned to the Earth. Once you can hold space for whatever you discover in your inner cosmos, you can transform these gems into anything that most supports your healing journey. As if you can visit that point along the river where a rock is damming the flow, recognize this blockage, remove the stone, and stand back as the waters flow freely. While every single chakra is part of the large cosmic orbit within the human body and every center is intertwined with the other, the second and the fifth chakra are intimately interwoven. A blockage in one will directly impact a blockage in the other. Likewise, clearing energy in one will directly affect an opening in the other.

The fifth chakra, represented by the color blue or teal, lives within your throat. This is where your authentic voice may be free to share itself with the world or where your vocal cords tighten as protective gatekeepers that interfere with your capacity to speak your truth. Any stories you may have created about your voice at a young age could still be stored in your subconscious and may impact how you move through your world as an adult. For example, perhaps you were told you were too loud as a child, so you stored a memory in your throat chakra that it was safer to be silent. Maybe you were shy and panicked whenever you needed to use your voice. Perhaps you spelled a word wrong in the spelling bee and felt shame in your throat. Maybe you raised your hand in class and proudly answered a math problem incorrectly. Perhaps you sang the wrong note in your school play.

What stories come up for you about the way that you related to your voice as a child?

Whatever wants to present itself to you, hold space to listen compassionately and release any judgments about what may arise. Something that perhaps you thought your entire life was the most insignificant little event may trigger a profoundly transformational emotional process for you in the present moment. Maybe this story or this emotion had been waiting all of this time to be recognized in a way your younger self could not hold.

My Vocal Transformation mentor, Maryn Azoff, explains that when all of our chakras are balanced, especially the throat chakra, you no longer need to talk down; instead, you are free to speak up. This means you no longer need to engage in self-deprecating or violent language toward yourself or another. Instead, you project from your open heart, sharing compassion and forgiveness when you speak. You become open to sharing your truth with yourself and another, calling them to rise instead of trying to bring them down.

If your throat chakra is blocked, you may feel anxious about speaking in public, asking for what you need, singing, making requests, and having difficult conversations. When your throat chakra is balanced, you can think and verbalize positive and loving affirmations toward yourself and others. You take pleasure in using your voice in a mindful and liberated way. You know your truth, and feel free to express it. Acknowledging that the vulva, vocal cords, pelvic floor, jaw, and uterus are all in an intimate dance can free you to explore healing medicines that may balance either chakra and witness the magic flow freely through your being.

If you notice that your throat feels closed and are having difficulties singing or speaking, it may support you to circle your hips and engage in sensual circular movement of the pelvic floor. Likewise, if you are feeling womb pain or imbalance in your sexual creative energy, it may support you to sing, scream, massage your throat, and wiggle out the tension in your jaw.

In my practice, hula hooping has been and continues to be a sacred medicine for liberating my womb space through cyclical spiral movement. As I rock my hips, I also support the free expression of my voice. The most profound medicine for my holistic wellness and healing journey has been connecting to my voice as a medicine tool for my liberation.

When you sing, you are re-patterning any stories you have created about whether your voice is "good" or "bad." When you sing, you allow the energy of creation to flow through your being by opening your throat to divine music. So whether you hum, chant a mantra, make up a song, or sing along to your favorite music, you support the liberation of your authentic voice. Let go of any expectation of how you think your voice should sound. Release any attachments to your voice sounding like anyone else's. This is about you sharing your unique, divine voice with this world.

You may wonder what singing in the shower has to do with feeling the courage to ask your partner for what you want sexually. You may wonder what chanting a mantra has to do with having the courage to ask your boss for the raise you feel you deserve. You may wonder what circling your hips has to do with releasing the tension in your jaw. They have everything to do with each other. As you may have noticed throughout this book, there are infinite opportunities to notice overlapping cyclical mandalas within and around you. Everything is interconnected, and many systems can serve as microcosms for larger processes that need to spiral through your emotional body.

My invitation to you is to liberate your voice through sacred song. Feel free to learn some of your favorite songs and belt them freely, or put them aside and make up your own. Feel free to sing alone or gather your friends for a co-created song circle. Feel free to sing the wrong note or lyric and release any sound that may be authentic to you. We use our voice as a healing tool, so the point is liberation, not sounding pretty.

Your voice is worthy of being heard.

Your story is worthy of being shared.

Stories

To Be The Breath of Harmony

At this moment, I am lacking absolutely nothing. I couldn't be more grateful for the abundance and magic surrounding me.

I live in a beautiful clay house where I can open my window and harvest avocados. I can always hear the song of the rushing crystalline river below, like a clearing energy flowing infinitely. The desert-like rocky mountains surround this Peruvian valley with its barren sand and endless water. I have never seen mountains without a single shrub growing on its face, but there is something about these sacred apus that makes me feel completely protected and cared for. The river travels down the snow-capped mountains, a six-hour winding drive to its source. This is, of course, how long it would take for a human to get from our river spot to the source up the mountain, but I wonder how long it takes for water to travel down the river from its sacred home at over 10,000 feet elevation to the river that borders our land.

After spending one year traveling around different permaculture communities in Colombia and Ecuador, I arrived at this beautiful oasis three hours southeast of Lima. Although I came as just another volunteer, the permanent residents, four men, quickly absorbed me into their inner circle and offered me an opportunity to live with them long-term. It has been healing to notice how much I have grown and ascended in my spiral so that the opportunities I am presented with match this trusting, confident, rejuvenated part of me. Yes, I found myself arriving at a place with a strong masculine energy, but these were not men who aimed to take advantage of my soft feminine. They were strong, healthy, balanced brothers who truly sought to support me and uplift the feminine beauty within.

Upon arriving, I felt ecstatic and humbled to receive an opportunity to bury my *mochila* backpack for a little while. Was it possible that just from the medicine that I carried and the light that this community saw in me, I could live in my own clay home by the river, participate in retreats, eat delicious food, and not need to exchange a single penny for it all? I felt I had arrived in a dreamland where I was given the gift to sink deeper into my calling as a medicine woman. With so much masculine energy in the space, I naturally sunk into a soft feminine role that was entirely new for me. Of course, I loved being feminine, but my experience on previous farms involved challenging physical labor, and to keep up, I had to step into my tough, action-oriented masculine. But in this space, the men 100% had my back on all the heavy-duty tasks, and of course, I was invited to participate in these tasks whenever I felt called. Still, I was never obligated to climb onto a roof and hammer or carry heavy bags of rocks if I didn't feel up to it. I could trust that the rest of my community was doing what they loved most, and I was free to choose what I loved most.

Spirit was calling me to be the breath of harmony within the space. Some days, I would build Earth altars around the land, pick flowers, reorganize the kitchen, and smudge the rooms with purifying incense. And I often spent many hours in the kitchen making sprouts, soaking seeds, fermenting kombucha, brewing ginger beer, and massaging pounds of cabbage to make our homemade sauerkraut. I was called to trust deeper in the men in the community who held me and remember that my simple presence was enough. I did not need to do or be anything to be worth it or accepted.

I learned this lesson the hard way when I took a few days away from the community to go into Lima and make money by playing music on the buses. I had spent an entire day singing with my ukelele, always beginning and ending with the same speech. "Hello, everyone. Good day. I hope you are well. I have come to share some live music with you all. I hope you enjoy… [insert the same two songs I usually sang on repeat on every bus]…. Thank you so much for listening. I want to share that I am an artist and a traveler, so if you would be willing to contribute in any way—applause, a smile, a coin—I would be eternally grateful. Have a great day!"

I was feeling exhausted and ready to rest. Instead of listening to my body and simply taking a bus home, I decided to push my limits a bit further. I had just finished playing a few songs on a bus, and my hands were full of coins. When I went to exit the bus, my hand got stuck in the door handle. My body stepped onto the pavement, and the bus began to drive away with my hand. I instantly screamed and dropped all of the coins onto the floor. The bus came to a halt and I maneuvered my crippled hand out of the handle and then the bus drove away. I began sobbing intensely, feeling emotionally traumatized, shocked, vulnerable, and in intense physical pain.

I knew that the owner of the permaculture project I currently called home was also in Lima and that I should probably call him for help. Yet I was in shock and couldn't figure out how to take the next steps. I was staying at a hostel with several other people and knew my body needed to cry. Whether I went back to the hostel to cry or cried on the streets, I knew I didn't have a quiet space to cry alone, so I just remained seated on the sidewalk crying for a long while, cradling my injured hand like a baby. Many people walked by and left plastic water bottles at my feet. I wanted to tell them that plastic was not a solution to anything, but I couldn't speak, and I knew that their intentions were kind.

Eventually, a man in business attire approached me and sat beside me. He asked how he could support me. He insisted on taking me to a hospital. At first, I felt hesitant because I have a general distrust of the Western medical system, and I also had no traveler's insurance. He told me not to worry about the financial implications of treatment. He was willing to cover the costs. I felt weary about receiving such generous help from a stranger, yet I also felt he arrived as my angel. So, I ultimately agreed to accept his help. He called the taxi, directed us toward a medical center, paid for the X-rays, and then headed on his way.

I somehow hadn't broken anything. I just had severe sprains and internal bruising. I was prescribed complete immobility for the next six weeks.

I felt like an extremely sensitive chord had been struck within me. What would happen if I couldn't use my hand for a while? I definitely couldn't do most farm jobs or even cook well. I felt a deep fear of abandonment and rejection arise. The voice of humility within me knew that I needed help, so I called upon the community member I knew was in Lima.

This brother accompanied me back to our community in the mountains and assured me that I could take this time to retreat, to rest, to heal and that they would all take care of me. I noticed then how hard it was for me to fully receive care and nourishment when it came to me. I loved to be the independent woman who always could carry on her own, and this inner strength had indeed served me in many moments when I needed it, but in this moment, I could lean into the support around me. My simple existence was worthy of love, even if I couldn't give back in all the ways I would have liked.

Over time, I recovered the use of my hand and slipped back into a new role within the community, finding the balance between the soft feminine energy within as well as my strong, action-oriented masculine. I took so much pleasure in embodying the range of female archetypes to my fullest, feeling supported to show up in my authentic ebbs and flows and to communicate in each phase of my cycle.

This was the first time I began to claim one or two days in complete solitude when my moon came. My space and silence were always respected. The community recognized that taking space for my moon ritual was essential to my overall health and well-being as a cyclical woman.

Throughout my time, I was encouraged to sing and share my medicine music and after long months of playing on the streets for money, it felt supportive to play to the mountains, the river, for myself, and for my community. When groups rolled in for retreats, I loved picking flowers and smudging everyone upon arrival as they shed some of the city's heaviness and let it all ascend into sacred smoke.

We are in the middle of a permaculture design course, and everyone from our gathering nominated me to coordinate our last night's goodbye party celebration! In me, they see a fertile woman vibrating with happiness and enjoying her life. And seeing myself through that reflection, I remember that I am that woman. I am free to embody this joy and expand it outwardly fully. I am allowed to experience connection and continue opening my heart. In this moment of my moon cycle, I feel so much compassionate love glowing in my heart and pulsating through my whole being. Thank you, Great Spirit, for guiding me to this beautiful home in this present moment.

Braiding Chamomile Into Our Hair

Spring in Argentina is a magical time. After having lived through my first real bone-chilling cold winter, warmth was returning to the land. Yesterday, November 11, 2019, I woke at 4 a.m., buzzing with positive energy and excitement to express my creativity. I had just finished bleeding one day prior and awoke to the sensation of rebirth and rejuvenation within my body. I opened the zipper of my tent and sat in the hammock hanging from the tree that created the only shady spot in this expansive prairie. I had a few hours of cool dawn weather before the sun took its place in the sky and began shining his potent, warm rays on the land.

I wrote in my journal. I took my time preparing a slow breakfast. I drank mate, played my ukulele, and sang. Then, at 10 a.m., a dear friend surprised me under my tree. It is always a gift to be in this graceful woman's presence. She embodies her feminine beauty with delicacy, softness, and poise. She reminds me to pause and pick flowers. She reminds me how joyful it is to dress up our body temples by braiding each other's hair and painting our lips with a slight touch of gloss. She reminds me to carry essential oil wherever I go so I may share herbal medicines with the people I love. She reminds me to add a pinch of sugar into any savory dish we create and a pinch of salt into any sweet culinary creation so that we may bring life to our dishes. She reminds me that it is okay to ask for help and lean into the love of those around us.

We spent the day in a flirty trance together until it was time to leave our home in El Campo (a plot of land two hours south of Buenos Aires) so that we could attend our contact improvisation class. We began our long trek toward the bus stop, walking at a pace as if we had nowhere else to be but the present moment. We stopped to pick wild chamomile flowers that grew in fields by the acre, planted by none other than the wisdom of the Pachamama in springtime. We braided the flowers into our hair and stuffed them in our backpacks to sprinkle into our mates later. We picked and filled our bellies with infinite November *moras* (mulberries) from the pregnant purple trees we found along the way. When we found a cool, shady cove of trees thick with moisture and mosquitos, we rested in this refuge from the blazing sun. Here, we entered into a slow, sensual contact dance. I felt that we could have danced amongst the trees for hours. But eventually, we picked up our bags and continued our dance toward the bus stop.

When we finally arrived at the bus stop, we waited 20 minutes for the bus to take us to the train station. The train left every hour, so when our bus pulled up to the station, and we saw that the train was about to leave, we sprinted off of the bus and jumped right over the turnstiles as we always did and exhaled a breath of relief to have made it onto the train. When we were close to arriving at our stop, we noticed that we were already late and had 15 minutes of walking from where the train left us to our class. Our teacher could not stand for anyone arriving late to class. So we decided to run like cheetahs for eight blocks until we sprinted through the door of our class, completely winded. When we arrived, everyone was blindfolded and rolling around on the floor. We quickly dropped our bags, caught our breath, avoided the disapproving glance from our teacher, made our way down to the ground, blindfolded ourselves, and began rolling with the group.

I found myself in an incredible dance with this woman whom I always connected with through pleasurable liquid-like spirals. We both had our eyes blindfolded, so from our shared pelvic center, we took deep breaths and used each other's bodies as the Earth. We did not need to see each other; it was as if we were guided by eyes on our pelvis and instantly gravitated toward each other's center. We also poured our weight into the ground and kept rolling, giving, and receiving weight from our shared center.

I felt that this dynamic opened up the possibility for the rest of the class to flow in such a fluid, effortless way, and even when the class finished, I continued rolling in one fluid motion into the jam, where I also had incredible dances. Contact jams are open improvised movement spaces where we typically dance without music and are free to flow in and out of contact with others as we engage in non-verbal conversations with our own bodies and each other.

I had my first dance with this man with whom I have always wanted to dance. I feel that he moves in a way that is always deeply listening in whatever duo he may be in, and he brings a playful, slightly sexual energy into all of his dances. I am unsure if he perceived something similar in our micro dance, but these were some of the things I experienced within my body throughout our dance. He was lying face up, in an open star expansive position, and I began to roll closer to him. I placed my head on his arm, and we connected our parallel centers. I felt my heartbeat accelerate as we lay together in stillness for a few breaths, sensing each other. In a shared inhale, he scooped me toward him, and we began rolling together super slowly and sensually until we naturally arrived at a pause. Once again, he lay in an expansive position face up, and my body lay perpendicularly on top of him with my uterus over his solar plexus. He rested his hands on my lower back, inviting me to sink deeper into his center.

We took deep, synchronized breaths, and I felt so much heat circling through our shared center. My uterus and vaginal canal pulsated strongly, and I visualized myself releasing any tension through our shared breath. I felt that I was beginning to have micro orgasms through our touch, heat, visualizations, and synchronized respiration. I felt deeply embodied pleasure. From far away, we may have looked like one body lying on top of another. Yet, from close, I felt infinite waves of small orgasms dancing in our bodies. When we naturally began to move together again, we arrived at another pause where I was lying face up, and he was lying perpendicularly over my pubis bone. That exact placement caused me some pain, so I used my hands to roll him up a bit higher toward my chest, and we ended up with his penis resting right over my heart. We breathed together for a while, and I felt contractions and pulsations throughout my whole body, my uterus, my vaginal canal, my heart, our shared center, my hands, and his penis.

We kept our dance in a slow rhythm for an extended time until, naturally, the energy escalated, and we began spiraling faster and inhabiting higher levels. In one spiral toward the sky, I lifted him, and on the way down, we collided into another duo. Within a matter of breaths, two twos became four, became a new set of twos. We exchanged a glance as if to thank each other for the profound quality of that dance and then sank back into our new duo. It felt as if I wasn't beginning a new dance but instead continuing a dance that had already been alive in me for hours.

I was hypnotized by the movement of two beautiful women dancing in each other's space without entering into contact. As I witnessed their movement, my body began to join in their empty spaces, and the three of us began to dance together in such an organic way without bringing our bodies close enough to touch each other's skin, yet simply observing the movement of the other and allowing them to influence our movements. As we moved, we began to circulate a beautiful triangular energy. Then, naturally, the spaces between our bodies became smaller, and we started dancing contact in a trio on the ground on our hands and knees. We moved with such playful energy, in a flirty way, like animals. I felt how whole-heartedly we could each connect to the curious little girls within us and allow this innocence to guide our exploration.

Our trio was flowing incredibly, and in one moment, my friend joined in, and we slowly began to move as a quartet. We moved together as a foursome until we danced into two separate duos. I was in a super sensual, affectionate, pleasurable, and feminine dance with this beautiful woman with large eyes and long hair. We lost ourselves deeply in the dance, and sometimes, we would cross paths with the other duo and continue to flow together.

In one moment, the four of us paused in the center, surrendered into the ground, hugging each other, breathing together. I closed my eyes and felt we were just one organism with four extremities and one central breath. I felt a deep exhale embrace my entire being and body. At that moment, I felt I did not need anything, simply allowing the profound calmness to wash through my being. Of course, thoughts would arrive, and just as they entered, they would float by like clouds. We sighed deeply together, and I felt collective surrender, support, trust, openness, and pleasure. I began to hum a soft melody and found myself singing with the other woman with whom I had not yet entered into a dance. I felt that our voices joined a powerful dance. She was the Earth, singing the deeper base notes. I flew over her solid ground. Together, our voices took flight, and our entire organism of four bodies flew as well.

Mujer Volcan, Volcano Woman

After spending nearly a year dancing in Buenos Aires and having already hopped over to Uruguay twice for a quick border run that would renew my visa, I felt curious to explore a new border as my three months were close to expiring again.

The blazing hot summer was raging through the city, and most of my friends were getting ready to leave the heavy humidity for a few months and return in the Fall. A few weeks before I was set to leave, I connected in a deliciously unexpected, intimate way with a beautiful Chilean woman. She and I had been a part of a queer collective of women-only contact dancers for the last year and had spent many hours dancing, rolling, and chatting together. So, one day, she visited our contact family in El Campo and spent the night with us.

Eventually, everyone wandered off to bed except for her and me. I asked if she would like to come to my tent and smoke some ganja with me. Once we were together, slightly stoned in the tent, illuminated by a small candle, we began to let our bodies talk. We started with a slow, sensual dance of our fingertips until we rolled around together amongst the entangled blankets. If this had been a contact jam, there would be certain guidelines that the collective respects and agrees upon. At a jam, we all hold ourselves accountable to keep our dances *dances* and to put all other sexual energy to the side. Yes, touch is sensual and intimate, but in a jam, we don't cross the fine line into sexual exploration. However, this wasn't a jam; the only ones holding the container were the two of us and the expansive night sky. I began to perceive that the rolling and caressing was taking on an energy of direct flirtation and seduction. I felt her and I becoming aroused. She would take her time on each roll, finding ways to straddle me to stimulate the sensitive skin between her legs.

She was unapologetically moving in ways that would bring her into a deeper state of pleasure and laughing it off with an innocent smile when we would make eye contact. After much sweaty rolling, I had pinned her down below me, and I felt drawn to bring my face to her chest. Up until then, we hadn't explicitly crossed any sexual lines, but I felt a strong desire to begin kissing her chest.

I grabbed the edge of her shirt and motioned as if I wanted to take it off. I looked at her and asked, "*Puedo*? May I?" She responded, "*Podí hacer lo que tu queráis*... You can do whatever you want," with a mischievous smile. We spiraled into making beautiful, passionate, intensely sweaty love and came out of the tent hours later, naked, searching for fresh air. She came behind me and surprised me by rolling an icy cold water bottle down my back. The sensation of my hot, sticky body with the cool chill of the ice sent shivers down my spine. We fell asleep cuddled into each other, and the next day, we took her to the bus stop so she could return to the city.

We said see you soon because we would meet again in a few days at our weekly contact class and jam. I felt a bit nervous about our next meet-up, *reencuentro*, as I was traumatized by several times having shared in a powerfully intimate sexual exchange with a man, and upon seeing each other again, he would act standoffish, pretending as if nothing had occurred between us. I was pleasantly surprised to arrive at the jam and see that she had picked fresh jasmine flowers for me. We were both unintentionally dressed as twins, wearing the same black pants and green t-shirt. We danced in such a tender way, excited to hold each other again, and we also remained open to continue dancing with others. The way we showed up for each other at the jam brought such profound healing and rewiring for me, feeling that I was worthy of creating intimacy with humans who would show up in integrity, respect, and care.

Since I lived in El Campo, two hours away from the city, I had to coordinate sleepovers somewhere in the city if I wanted to stay late. There was a jam that I wanted to go to at the end of the week, so I called her and asked if she was going and if I could sleep over at her house after. She said yes with clarity and excitement. Once again, making plans with someone so wholly disentangled, simple, and ready to say yes to our connection was healing. The jam went on for several hours, and I noticed myself beginning to doubt if she would arrive, but of course, she did.

When we finished dancing, it was late, and we were hungry. We walked through the empty city streets at night to discover that every restaurant was closed. We stumbled upon a pizzeria that appeared to be open, so we walked in. But all of the chairs were already on the table, and they were closing down. We had such a contagious buzz of flirtation and love lingering between us that magical things happened when we moved through the world together. We got on the good side of the worker closing up shop, and he agreed to serve us while he finished cleaning. We ordered Faina, a typical Buenos Aires pizzeria specialty that is a sort of pancake made of chickpea flour cut into the shape of a pizza slice. Then he even gifted us empanadas. We were full of gratitude and laughter, soaking each other up on our "first date."

She had short, dark-black hair and smooth, caramel skin. Her eyes were big and black, brightly shining whenever she smiled her giant smile, which she often did. She had grown up in a lower-class family in Santiago until she moved to Buenos Aires to study dance. She discovered incredible theater, circus, music, and dance programs free in the city. She sustained herself economically by sewing and selling reusable menstrual pads and making mouth-watering vegan Snickers with homemade peanut butter and date paste. These chocolates were irresistible, I think because we could taste her in them and savor her love.

We were making love the night of our "first date" in her bedroom. I was in this entirely vulnerable, surrendered state where every part of my being was one with the sensations of fully embodied pleasure. I felt myself coming closer to an orgasm in this fuzzy, delirious state... and then,

"BAM!"

The curtain rod draped over her bed fell directly onto me, pounding me hard in the center of my heart chakra. Instantly, everything stopped. First, I felt numbness. Then, I felt grief. I began to sob as I gently caressed the circle on my chest that immediately turned purple. I know that accidents happen to anyone at any time. But I took this one personally. Here I was, finally, in an intimate sexual exchange with a beautiful woman in which there were no penises involved. Then, this large phallic object falls onto me, violently penetrating my heart space. I felt trapped, as if the ghost of penetrating violence during sex would be something I'd never thoroughly shake off. It was a significant learning experience for both of us, expressing how we felt impacted without truly being able to blame each other or the curtain rod or anything. But that's a memory that sends a sharp blow to my heart each time I recall that sensation of being in a state of 100% trust and then instantly switching into a panic.

She and I continued sharing in an incredible duo until she was getting ready to go back to Santiago to visit her family for the holidays, and my visa was expiring. We knew we had to part ways momentarily, but we also felt the opportunity to cross paths again soon. So we said goodbye for now as she went to Santiago, and I ventured north of Argentina near Salta.

I stayed for a few days with my dear brother, with whom I had lived in the Peruvian community. Then, I began my wild hitchhiking journey to cross the border in the Chilean desert of Atacama. The first day, I spent eight hours only a thirty-minute walk from my brother's house, watching infinite cars pass me all day without stopping. Finally, a small, run-down vehicle pulled over. A man was driving in front with a woman, two children, and a lot of stuff in the back. This was a tiny car, but they pushed some of their things to the side and made room for me to get in. I asked where they were going, and they said to a nearby town that was only a 30-minute drive away. I had a long way to go to the border, but anything that led me in that direction felt like the right step. So I hopped in and shortly found myself in a beautiful valley with a large rocky river flowing through the center. I found a secluded campground right by the river, where I decided to spend the night since it was nearly dark. I might as well rest and recharge to try my hitchhiking luck again tomorrow.

The next morning, a sweet Dutch couple who had rented a nice car immediately picked me up! They advanced me about four hours in the right direction. On the way, we passed thick green jungles and the rainbow-colored desert mountains of Jujuy. They then dropped me off at a fork where our roads diverged. I was in the middle of the desert with no humans or shops in sight. I fervently prayed that I would not get stranded here, and shortly after, a giant truck pulled over for me. I asked where he was headed, and he said he was crossing the border. Yippee! So I jumped right in, and we continued our winding journey through a vast expanse of an endless one-way road across the desert. I couldn't believe that I had woken up at a river, driven through dense green jungles, multicolored mountains, and barren deserts, and now looked out the window at what appeared to be mountains of snow.

The "snow" was actually a salt flat. We drove through miles of boundless salt, and the truck driver even pulled over for me to take a picture and lick the salt.

We were only a few hours from the border, but the driver started nodding off into sleep and then would suddenly jerk himself awake. The more this went on, the more nervous I became. I tried talking loudly, telling stories, singing, bumping up the air conditioning, insisting that he pull over to stretch, serving mate, anything to keep him awake. But he just wanted to power on through to the border. Somehow, we arrived safely at the border, where we had to get out of the truck and go through the immigration office.

Here, I discovered that this wasn't a border you could cross on foot. You had to be registered with a form of transportation. The truck driver couldn't register me because he had to show his immigration papers to his company, and picking up gringa travelers along the way is probably not a part of his business contract. So the truck driver went on without me, and I went to stand by the border, hoping that I could convince some kind person in a car to help me cross. Although I had a sweet face and feminine white privilege, I couldn't get anyone to trust me. Car after car said no, questioning the motives of this young American girl stranded at the border in the desert. As the sun began setting, my nervousness kicked in.

This border was one of the most hostile landscapes I had ever visited. We were 5,000 meters in altitude in a barren desert in the middle of nowhere. When the sun shone in the day, I felt I could pass out from high elevation mixed with heat stroke. But when the afternoon wind began to blow, it felt like a post-apocalyptic hostile winter. The potent wind knocked over everything in its path, sending a violent chill into my bones. I quickly released any notion of crossing the border that day, as the border was closing and it was getting dark. So I looked around at the isolated immigration office surrounded by a vast expanse of desert. I couldn't pitch my tent because I would freeze to death at night, or the wind would crack the tent poles and send me flying. I asked the immigration officer where I could spend the night, and he told me to *golpear la puerta*, knock on the door of one of the two other clay huts in the area.

I approached the house and found a tiny, run-down, deteriorated home with an aloof lady "greeting me." I briefly explained that I was looking for a place to spend the night so that I could cross the border in the morning. She offered me a filthy-looking closet-sized room, one of the three rooms in the whole house. It had a bed with a blanket, which was essential to survive the night. I had nowhere else to go, so I agreed. I asked her if there was anywhere I could get some food since I hadn't eaten all day. She said the other clay hut was a *tienda*, a little store.

I tried to run as fast as I could from one clay hut to the next, fearing that the harsh wind would knock me over, and when I made it to the tienda, I remembered that we were in a desert, hundreds of miles in any direction from any major city. I don't know why I had expected to find some fruits or vegetables, but to my disappointment, everything was packaged and processed. I couldn't cook anything, so I needed something I could eat immediately and then rest. Nothing in that tienda had any real nutrition, so I settled on bread rolls that were so hard I had to dip them in water to get them down. I set my alarm super early, and the cold early morning wind ferociously blew when I woke.

I wanted to ensure I was the first at the border. Perhaps some cars had already lined up, waiting for the immigration officer to open his doors, and I could chat with them while the border opened. But for a long while, no one came. Slowly, cars kept rolling through, and no one wanted to take me.

As the hours rolled by, the immigration officer began to take pity on me, so he agreed to help me. Instead of me going up to the cars and asking for their support, the man with a badge and gun stopped the next car and said they could pass, but he insisted they take me across the border. In the car was a sweet, nervous-looking family who I learned was Peruvian. A mom and dad were in the front, and two young boys in the back. Just a humble family on vacation, now responsible for getting this random gringa girl across the border in a somewhat sketchy situation. They seemed doubtful, but I heard them pray aloud to Jesus. They asked for his protection and affirmed that they were doing this from the goodness of their hearts. Well, the officer used his position of power to support me, and with the help of this family, I made it through! They took me all the way to San Pedro de Atacama, where I was headed, and they carried on their journey back up to Peru.

Eventually, I returned to Santiago, where I reconnected with my lover from Buenos Aires. We made plans to travel together back to Buenos Aires. We agreed to hitchhike and camp along the way and made a pact to try to spend as much time as possible in fresh water. Finding water could have been a challenge as there are long stretches of monoculture Monsanto corn and soy fields in the flat expanse in the center of Argentina. But we managed to spend every night by a river or creek. We got rides from the most beautiful humans, friendly truck drivers, a dad traveling with his young child, and a generous lesbian couple. We spent a long while camping at the top of a mountain where a crystalline river flowed in the mountains of Cordoba. There, we met many unique travelers who had set up camp along the river, and we formed a loving community, cooking together by the fire and sharing songs.

Our time together was deeply healing as we relearned what it meant to be in a healthy partnership with someone.

Neither of us had ever felt so seen, safe, and held in an intimate relationship. So, we held space for shedding painful memories of past relationships and creating new memories of love, trust, freedom, and pleasure. Although our partnership did not last very long, the way we loved each other provided us an opportunity to rebirth, or in Spanish, *reverdecer* (meaning to become green again, like in the springtime.) We made our way back to Buenos Aires, and shortly after, it was time for me to board my plane back to California after three years in South America. She took me to the airport, where we hugged and kissed goodbye, saying, *"Nos vemos pronto,* See you soon."

I concluded that she was purely water and fire, which is why I began calling her Mujer Volcan, Volcan Woman. Eventually, I wrote her a song; below, you can read the original lyrics in Spanish and an English translation.

Mujer Volcan

Nadando fuera de mi, dentro de mi, dentro de ti
Tus aguas fluyen con mis aguas
Y la luz eterna de esa estrella fugaz
Y el olor a la noche iluminada
Juntas desde la muerte al renacer
Juntas hacia la cumbre a reverdecer
Juntas vibrando en el placer
Juntas yo soy tu hermosa primavera
Mujer volcan me sembrare en el calor de tu vientre
Mujer volcan fluiré por tus mareas del sentir
Mujer volcan me encenderé en tu rio de llamas

Volcano Woman

Swimming outside of myself, yet inside of myself, and inside of you
Your waters flow with my waters
And the eternal light of that shooting star
And the aroma of the illuminated night
Together from death to rebirth
Together to blossom at the peak of the mountain
Together vibrating in pleasure
Together, I am, your beautiful Springtime
Volcano woman, I will plant myself in the heat of your womb
Volcano woman, I will flow in your tides of emotion
Volcano woman, I will light myself ablaze in your river of flames

Clear Vision

Immediately upon graduating high school, I left my mother's home with a ravenous curiosity to explore the diversity and beauty of this Earth. I spent a year living in Israel, studying at a social justice-focused liberal arts college in California, and studying abroad in Ecuador. I backpacked for three years throughout Colombia, Ecuador, Peru, Chile, Argentina, and Uruguay. I always felt slightly ungrounded throughout my travels as this persistent call for rooting down into home kept making its way into the forefront of my visions and prayers. I knew I could visit my mother in Los Angeles and that she would gladly receive me in her home. Yet still, it was clear to me that this was not the territory I would choose to *hechar raíces*—put my roots into the soil. I met so many beautiful travelers on my journeys who loved the magic of *la ruta libre*, the free path. And they always knew they had a place they could return to during their travels.

Where and when would I feel that deeply relieving exhale that I had arrived at my community?

Even though I could not clearly see the "how" I would get there, the sensation of home and community was strikingly clear in my vision and the warmth of my heart.

When I finally decided to visit my mom for what I assumed would be a short grounding visit, the pandemic lockdown began within a couple of weeks. For me, this period, like for many, brought the energy of winter and hibernation. I knew that spring would come again, but first, I had to be present with the winter by really getting clear on where I would like to blossom in the coming phase. Many places on this Earth called out to me, places I had been to and some that I had yet to explore. Yet, more important than attaching to a specific place was clarifying my vision as sensations in my body, allowing myself to be surprised by the great mystery of life, allowing each step to unfold in divine perfection.

A year later, once the lockdown had eased, I found myself having taken an incredible step in the right direction toward a new, unexpected community in Northern California. This reminded me of my vision, and I knew I was close, yet my intuition told me, "Not yet. Enjoy the ride, but you're not home yet. It gets better. Yes, you can have everything you have dreamed of." While it was challenging to say goodbye, I felt deep gratitude for the medicine shared on those sacred lands and found myself journeying to Costa Rica.

Costa Rica was never part of my plan, but perhaps Spirit had other plans for me. I love the saying, "We plan, God laughs," reminding us how impossible it is to control our fates in the face of the great mystery. I released attachments to what form or structure my vision would take and surrendered deeply to trusting the process. I traveled to a few different parts of Costa Rica, and while I recognized the beauty of the breathtaking landscapes, I felt that this was not the place for me. I tried to open doors, seek community, take aligned action steps toward fulfilling my vision, and all of the doors kept closing for me before I could even walk through them. I felt this was Spirit's way of telling me to honor my no, close the door, and move on. There was no use in investing energy in converting what had felt like a clear no into a maybe or a yes. When something is a total yes for me, there's no way to deny it. Nothing is forced. It just flows effortlessly.

Although sometimes I felt hopeless, lost, alone, and vulnerable, I constantly renewed my faith through prayers and rituals. In one potent moon blood ritual in Costa Rica, I created my first medicine wheel with thirty-six stone offerings prayed for and set intentionally. I sat with my journal and guitar, and the song Clear Vision was born.

Clear Vision

I am singing my prayer for home and community
As I bleed from my sacred center back to the mother
As I see and I feel this clear vision in my heart
Where the crystalline rivers flow in infinite purity
Where children learn and play freely and wildly
Where elders share their wisdom and guide what we cannot see
Where we sit to heal and celebrate in sacred ceremony
Estoy elevando mi rezo pa sentirme ya en casa
Y en comunidad mientras sangro desde mi vientre sagrado
Te entrego mi luna a ti madre tierra
Y veo y siento esta clara visión en mi corazón
Where the womb keepers circle with the moon in prayer and magic
Where we shine our divine gifts and grow in intimate relationships
Where we tend to the soil in our garden and nourish our souls in abundance

Where sacred harmony is interwoven into the flower of
our life
Show me the way Great Spirit, *Muestrame Gran Espiritu*
Guide me Mother Earth, *Guiame Pachamama*
I am open to receive, *Estoy abierta a recibir*
I am trusting in the mystery, *Confiando en el misterio*
Where we co-create and birth music and dance and all
kinds of art
Where our expression is raw and true and radically honest
from our heart
Where life holds presence, playfulness, pleasure, and
purpose
Where we all have everything we need and more

With this clear vision, I knew I had to take the next step.
I debated between a few different places, and I felt a strong
pull to explore the magic of Lake Atitlan, Guatemala. There,
once again, I could recognize beauty. But my soul knew this
was not the place I would ever want to put roots down. If I
thought doors had been closed for me in Costa Rica, they
were slammed violently shut in my face in Guatemala. I had a
challenging time sustaining any intimate relationship, finding
work, and connecting with the Pachamama. I felt that the
stream's waters and the lake were pushing me far away. I
connected to a sense of heaviness within me around this
never-ending feeling of searching for a home and feeling out
of place. Yet, I continued trusting, feeling gratitude for each
step of the journey, and maintaining my vision. I felt there
was no use in investing energy into converting something
that felt like a clear no into a yes when I could simply close
the door and move toward my clear YES!
Months passed, and while I was sure to leave the lake
soon, I was waiting for a clear message on my direction. In

one shamanic drum journey I attended at the lake, I was guided to visualize a powerful place in nature. Instantly, I recalled this magical bridge that crossed a sparkling river in Vilcabamba, Ecuador. On the bridge, I met a *jaguar negro*, a black jaguar, and I connected to the infinite well of wild, untamed, fierce energy within me. I would have stayed lifetimes on that bridge growling with the jaguar, feeling bold and courageous. Still, I was guided to continue my visualization on a downward path, to keep going in deeper. The jaguar crossed the bridge to the other side of the river, and I followed him. He led me down to the water, where a beautiful mermaid awaited me. She motioned for me to get into the water, and although the river appeared shallow, I took a deep dive in. I pushed a large river rock to the side and began swimming deep into an ocean below the surface, following the mermaid through dark waters.

When I returned from this vision, I knew that the sacred waters of Vilcabamba were calling to me, and within a week, I closed my chapter at the lake and arrived in Ecuador. As soon as I arrived, I began receiving opportunities to accompany children in creative processes through play, nature, and art; to hold women's circle rooted in the magic of our moon cycle; to play live music in different settings and get paid in abundance; to sit in powerful ancestral healing ceremonies; to easily create and sustain intimate relationships; to move into my own home where I could live near the river, grow my own food, and elevate my prayers. I finally understood that Vilcabamba was where I was meant to be.

Of course, rooting down has not been easy. After over ten years of constant travel, I had developed some escapist tendencies. As soon as the honeymoon phase ended, I began clinging to the imperfections and creating suffering for myself. Yes, I know that there will never exist a perfect place and community. And truthfully, my vision isn't about finding that picture-perfect utopia. It's about finding a place and a group of people who want to do the work together.

As long as we can continue to show up in love and authenticity and feel nourished in reciprocity, the process is the most interesting bit, not the end goal. I constantly remind myself of this as I currently rent a humble mountain house with a giant garden, a kitchen with a view, and a fireplace. This is not the house of my visions at all. I continuously dream about building my home with clay, bamboo, and wood. Yet living here and now is like laying down an essential plank of the railway so that my vision may continue evolving smoothly along the tracks, one simple wooden plank at a time.

I have poured so much love into making this place a harmonious temple. I made offerings, held rituals, and planted hundreds of flowers and medicinal herbs. Right now, as I learn to care for this place, I trust that in divine timing, the perfect land and humans to weave with will step forward so that we may share our medicine in this valley. I dream about having a partner and stewarding a piece of land together throughout our lifetime and for generations to come. I dream of a giant circular gathering space with sleek wooden floors that serves as a space to hold retreats, medicine ceremonies, concerts, contact improvisation jams, and workshops surrounded by abundant fruit trees and a medicinal herb garden alongside the river. I am constantly reminded that I am in the perfect place at the ideal time, and each step is getting me closer and closer to fulfilling this vision. And meanwhile, I am learning and growing along the way.

Fully Embodied Fertility

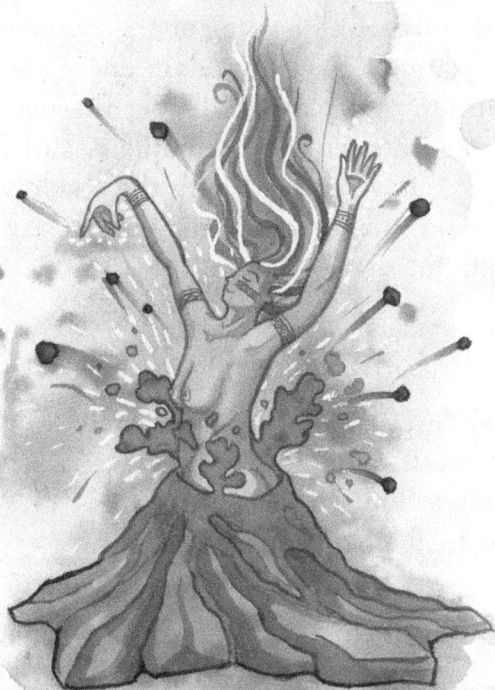

Moon's Energy

The moon is at its most fertile peak! This phase is a period of expansive luminous light with all the creative, fertile energy necessary to connect with your external environment. As the waters rise from the roots of every plant to its leaves and fruits, this is the best time to harvest and receive the full potency of the full moon's healing energy. Likewise, with this infinite light, you may have abundant energy to manifest the seeds of intention you planted during the new moon. This is a time to celebrate, connect, complete, and rejoice in the moon's light. We have danced with the shadows of the new moon and are now ready to dance our most radiant selves fully into the light.

Moon Phase: Full Moon

The Full Moon phase falls approximately on days 14-21 of the moon cycle. However, days before the full moon reaches its peak, you are sure to feel its potent effects on your body.

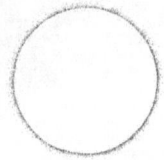

Menstrual Cycle Phase: Ovulation

In a bleeding body's menstrual cycle, this is the ovulation period. Since the end of your last menstrual cycle, your body has begun rebuilding and preparing a nourishing home within your uterus for potential life to start sprouting. Your ovaries release an egg that may be fertilized and create life. Since most ovulation days your egg is not fertilized, you release it and do not become pregnant. Although your energy may not be poured into creating a new life, you have an infinite well of abundant creative energy within you, ready to be poured into something. You may feel called to nourish a personal project or relationship or manifest a vision stored deep within your heart. Witness yourself in the full embodiment of its expression.

I tend to feel a deep need for social connection at this time and feel my heart and body bursting with compassion. There is plenty of energy within me to take care of and nurture myself and also to take care of others. I also feel that, at this time, I am unapologetically expressive. I love to take up a lot of space, and I want others to witness my beauty, confidence, and creative expression.

Cervical Dance

Fertile cervical fluids are designed to trap sperm within the womb to promote egg fertilization. So your fluids may be extra sticky, slinky, slimy, clear, or egg whitey. These days, avoid penis-in-vagina sex if you are not looking to conceive. Alternatively, this fertile window is the best time to have penis-in-vagina sex if you want to conceive. It is impossible to precisely say what days of your menstrual cycle this will fall on since all bodies are different, and individual cycles will vary monthly. By tracking your cycle and noticing your fertile cervical fluid, you can become autonomous over your reproductive health and make conscious, natural choices about your conception desires.

If you are tracking your basal body temperature as a fertility marker, you can only confirm ovulation after you have ovulated by noticing a higher temperature the following morning. So, if you feel you may be ovulating, you can lean into signs from your body like increased energy, increased arousal, and fertile cervical fluids. If you have been checking your cervix throughout your cycle, in this fertile window, it will be high and soft (ideal for sperm to travel upward).

Season: Summer

This is the season of Summer, when all the tomatoes, peaches, basil, cucumbers, and cantaloupes decide to have a party and fruit in abundance all simultaneously. These are the longest days of the year in which we are constantly nourished by the life force energy of the Great Father Sun, Taita Inti. Perhaps summer reminds us of the scent of late-night bonfires on warm nights, the taste of salty waves on our lips from long days at the beach, or the dribbling juices of a refreshing watermelon running down our chin. This is our time to shine without holding anything back. The energy of the summer season invites us into an outward expression of connection and celebration. As we soak up reserves of Vitamin D for the winter and fill our hearts with juicy social connections, we embody the feeling of having arrived at the mountain's peak and enjoy the view with deep gratitude.

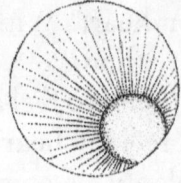

Element: Fire

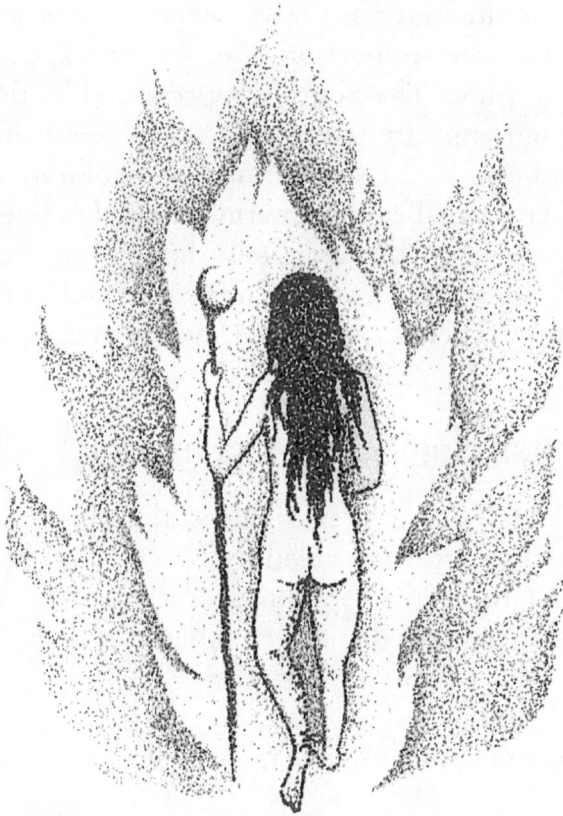

This phase is the Fire Element, representing expansive, passionate, transformational medicine. If you have the opportunity to gather by a fire on the Full Moon, invite your friends and bring offerings and prayers. You can pray for something you would like support in manifesting and something you would like to release and let go. With the heat of the fire, you are nourished as you watch your prayers ascend directly toward the creator in sacred smoke.

Direction: South

This is the direction of the South, represented by the color Red. We are invited into our most radiant power and inner strength, feeling the support of all of our ancestors holding space for us to shine. The South is represented by the snake, symbolizing our capacity to transmute and change our skin. Snakes have been used cross-culturally to connote wisdom, fertility, and creative life force energy. Kundalini yoga allows you to snake energy through your body from your root chakra up through your crown. This process can unfold with the help of the serpent as you shed the old and embody the new.

Astrological Signs: Fire Signs

Aries: Aries is the first sign of the Zodiac, a cardinal fire sign ruled by Mars, often referred to as the Big Bang. Aries energy can be chaotic, dispersed, intense, passionate, and excited. This powerful, enthusiastic portal is for creating new projects and connecting to your inner ambition.

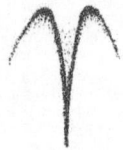

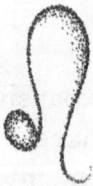

Leo: Leo is the fifth Zodiac and second fire sign, a fixed sign ruled by the Sun. While the fire of Aries is a wild cannon of infinite potential energy, the fire of Leo is much more egotistical and centered on an "I" experience. This is a powerful time to embody radical selfishness, tuning into your deepest heart's desires and sharing them unapologetically with the world. Leo's energy can manifest as feeling misunderstood, dramatic expression, and a fully embodied expression of fearless love for oneself and others.

Sagittarius: Sagittarius is the ninth sign of the Zodiac, the third and final fire sign, and a mutable sign ruled by Jupiter. While Leo's fire energy concerns self, this is a socially extroverted connective fire. Sagittarius's energy is focused, playful, enthusiastic, and humorous. This is a powerful portal to test your fortune, aim your arrow directly toward something you wish to manifest, and easefully allow the magic to unfold.

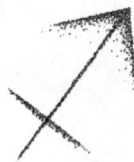

Female Archetype: Sensual Goddess & Mother

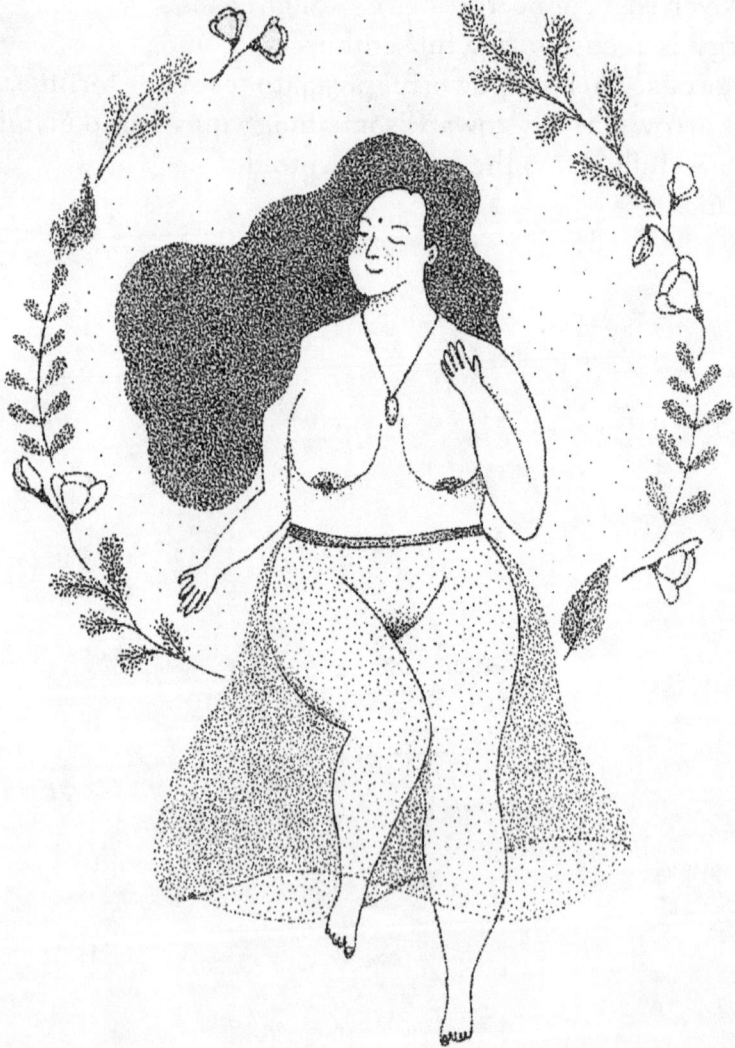

This phase is the archetype of the mother and sensual goddess. As you ovulate, you connect to loving, motherly, caretaking energy and the wild, sexually expressive goddess within you. You can take this time to reconnect to your mother, your lineage, the Great Mother Earth, and your mother within. Your hormonal shifts in this phase support your blossoming into compassionate, tender motherhood. Your physical body may slightly shift in appearance to signal to other potential mates that you are a safe place to implant their seed. Your breasts may become fuller, and your complexion rosier because you are stepping into your most empowered, sexy goddess.

It is through sex that all humans on this Earth were created. While society has deemed sex taboo, shameful, or secretive, it is truly an opportunity to connect to the source of your creative life force energy. So, if you aren't looking to conceive now, this may be a beautiful moment to go out on a date and channel your flirtatious energy. Or perhaps you have space to nurture a friend who could use your support lovingly. Or maybe you are curious about exploring a more profound self-pleasure practice. This phase can seem intense and overwhelming with so much creative potential available. Hold space to express whatever is alive in you during this time and release all judgments or expectations.

Suggested Foods

Essential nutrients that support your body in the ovulatory phase include zinc, antioxidants, fiber, omega-3, and B-12. Foods like pumpkin seeds, almonds, and oats contain zinc, which supports your body's rising testosterone levels. Flax seeds, a rich source of fiber and omega-3, support your body in metabolizing extra estrogen. Antioxidant-rich foods like broccoli and berries help decrease inflammation in the body to prevent premenstrual bloating. When your body receives raw or sprouted broccoli, it interprets this incoming information as a toxin. So, in response to this broccoli, your body produces a powerful antioxidant, Nrf2, which has healing effects on your entire body. Since testosterone and cortisol are highest in this phase, this can cause increased anxiety levels, depleting the body's magnesium. Luckily, one of the highest sources of naturally occurring magnesium in nature is found in cacao, so this is a perfect time to indulge in chocolate medicine.

Suggested Movement Plan

You may find that this is your most active time of the month. With increased testosterone levels, your body can support your most challenging workouts. So perhaps you can try a high-intensity interval training workout, acrobatics, hooping, or skating. This is also a great phase to try new body movements since you will have the endurance to practice in a playful and self-compassionate way throughout your cycle.

I genuinely feel that when ovulating, I have enough energy to take pleasure in my active body in its flow. And I know this is only possible because I deeply rested during my bleed. They almost seem like two different humans altogether. The one who can barely stop weeping enough to get out of bed and make herself a cup of tea. And the one who cleaned the kitchen, worked out, made love to herself, and wrote a chapter of her book all before 8 a.m. Yet the beauty is that both of these are me in different phases of my cycle. So, while it can be wild to ride along these cyclical waves, I have found that the most healing path of least resistance is to flow with the waves instead of forcing my body to act out of integrity with its natural rhythm.

So allow yourself to dance into your wildest, most active, energetic self in this phase, and don't hold anything back.

Fully Embodied Fertility

If you don't feel active or enlivened during ovulation for whatever reason, this is also okay, which is why I encourage you to track your cycle so you can best work with your flow! Release your expectations about how you think you should feel now, and listen to your womb. She'll tell you what she needs.

Suggested Herbal Support

I suggest working with Rose Petals, Cacao, Hibiscus, and other heart-opening herbs to sink deeper into this full moon magic. To soothe your internal waters, you can also try demulsifying herbs such as Slippery Elm and Marshmallow Root. These herbs may also stimulate cervical fluid production and can increase your sensation of vaginal wetness. You can take these herbs as a tea, tincture, herbal salve, or even drop some into an herbal bath.

Cyclical Gardening

The full moon is the time of the harvest. The water within each plant has risen to the fruits and leaves. No wonder a peach tastes juiciest on the full moon. This is a great phase to harvest medicinal herbs from your garden since the plant's medicine is concentrated in its leaves. While picking fresh herbs throughout the moon cycle is nourishing, you may want to harvest plenty of herbs during the full moon phase and let them dry so that you can access their medicine throughout the cycle until the next full moon. Enjoy harvesting from the fruits you planted during the new moon or perhaps many moons ago.

Alternatively, this is the best phase to pull out any weeds you would not like to grow in your garden. "Weeds" are incredibly strong and resilient. No human being planted them. They carry within their genetic material the wisdom to reproduce even in the harshest conditions. It's no wonder so many plants we consider weeds are incredibly medicinal. It's nothing short of a miracle that a plant can grow and thrive from a seed blown by the wind, perhaps in between cement cracks, rocks, or barren compacted soil. So maybe some incredibly medicinal weeds are growing in your garden bed, like stinging nettle, dandelion, and plantain. While honoring their medicine, there is also a time and place for weeds since they tend to be invasive. So if you weed on the full moon, since the plant's energy is up in its leaves, it will be weakened with much less likelihood that it will grow back, even if you don't entirely pull out the root. If you weed on the new moon, since the plant's roots are the strongest of the lunar phase, even if you think you completely pulled out the plant, just by leaving the tiniest little root in the soil, the weed will find a way to keep growing. The moon will tell you what your garden needs throughout her phases, how to tend to the soil and work with her rhythms as she waxes and wanes.

Writing Reflections

⟩ Is there a creative project that wants to be birthed through you right now?

⟩ What do you need to feel safe to sink into the pleasure of your creation process fully?

⟩ What personal pleasure practice can you cultivate within yourself to express your sensuality?

⟩ Are there any resistances that may arise for you around embodying the caretaking mother archetype?

⟩ Are there any resistances that may arise for you around embodying the sensual sexy goddess archetype?

⟩ What part of you is yearning to be seen, witnessed, and acknowledged by others?

☽ What can you give thanks to in this present moment, knowing that for many moons you had prayed for these things and are now harvesting in abundance?

Ovulatory Heart Opening Cacao Ritual

Cacao is the medicine of the heart and has been used to bring families, friends, and lovers together in the frequency of love for thousands of years. Cross-culturally, native wisdom has constantly returned to cacao medicine as a sacred heart opener. In Colombia and other countries in Central America, every home will have a *chocolatera*, a special vessel in which the cacao is prepared, representing the feminine ability to contain. The cacao is mixed with a special phallic stick called a *molinillo*, representing the masculine quality to penetrate. In this way, the cacao is prepared through the sacred union of the masculine and feminine, merging their essences into one, blossoming into deeper love. So, with every intentional cup of cacao you drink, you bring balance to the feminine and masculine energies within you.

Cacao is rich in magnesium, theobromine, and many other vitamins and minerals that support your body to feel good. The theobromine increases serotonin and dopamine within your body, which creates an elated feeling of joy, pleasure, and connection.

Traditionally, cacao was prepared by the women of the household, and this was an opportunity for them to pour their prayers into the Mama Cacao. So, in your ovulatory days, when your heart is most open and emanating fertile light, you have the potential to brew up a potent pot of cacao and watch the magic unfold. Cacao is also an aphrodisiac, so it is the perfect medicine to weave into your lovemaking.

If you have never ceremonially worked with cacao, I want to share my experience with this medicine. When

I first began my travels in Colombia, I somehow received an intuitive message to go toward a small town, San Gil. Although no one I knew had ever been there, I heard that there was a giant river, waterfalls, and mountains. And for me, it is always a step in the right direction wherever sweet water flows in abundance. So, when I arrived at the town center, I began asking around for places where I could camp or where I could be near the river. Unfortunately, I wasn't getting any answers that worked for me. While there was access to a large beautiful river within walking distance from the town center, most visitors stayed in hotels and private cabins. This was not the type of experience I was looking for.

I continued asking around but did not find much luck until I saw a painting of a giant jaguar and a huge dream catcher hanging inside a nearby hallway. I didn't know what the place was, but something about it called me in. I discovered it was a hostel, and I began conversing with the owner, explaining what I was looking for and asking if he had any leads. He told me his friends owned a beautiful permaculture cacao and coffee farm about 45 minutes up the mountain. They were getting ready to offer a natural building course with bamboo, so they would probably be happy to receive a helping hand. My whole body instantly felt it was a total yes, so I gave them a call, but I got no answer. I waited a bit longer and tried calling again, but still no response. I decided to go straight there since I had nowhere else to go, and this seemed like my most interesting lead. The hostel man told me they probably preferred I check in with them first, but still, he gave me directions on how to get there.

I had to hop on a little minivan that would take me up the mountain, and of course, as soon as we got inside the van, it began pouring rain, like a real tropical rain beating down ferociously. I knew the little bus would drop me off at a footpath about a thirty-minute walk from the farm. When I finally arrived at the point, I dashed to "shelter" under a tree, but I was already getting soaked. I felt I had no choice but to power through the rain and reach my destination. I had a giant backpack behind me, a smaller backpack in front of me, and a ukulele swung over my shoulder that I tried to keep dry with a plastic trash bag. The rain poured with vehemence while I continued following the dirt trail.

I finally saw a beautiful woven mandala hanging in the distance, and I felt that this had to be the place. I picked up my pace and arrived at a gate. I began to yell loudly, attempting to make my voice audible over the thundering rain. I shouted *unos saludos*, a few greetings, before a human appeared. He ran toward the gate with a big umbrella and quickly opened it for me. I followed him toward the house, where I unloaded my soaking wet belongings and exhaled deeply.

The man briefly disappeared and returned with warm tea and a banana. He asked if I had eaten lunch yet, and I said no. Together, we walked into the kitchen where two humans were making tamales, and they asked if I wanted to help. I couldn't believe that even though no one was expecting me or knew who I was or my intentions, they were so lovingly willing to receive me with open arms and invite me into their home. After preparing a meal together, we sat down for lunch, and I finally felt a need to know a bit more about where I had landed. It turns out that they were a permaculture farm that typically received volunteers. Although they were accustomed to being notified beforehand, they believed that the Great Spirit guided them and constantly sent them the medicine and messages their souls needed.

I fell deeply in love with these sacred lands where a mountainous, lush, wet jungle thrived in abundance amongst coffee, cacao, bananas, yuccas, papayas, and mangos. As the moon entered its waxing phase, I learned to prepare for the upcoming cacao harvest. One night, I entered the forest, guided by the full moon's light. I carried a giant bucket strapped around my shoulder to bring the cacao fruits back home. Each time I arrived at a tree, I learned to present myself and ask for permission to harvest from her fruits. I explained that my intentions were to take her seeds and create sacred heart medicine. At some trees, I offered tobacco, sang a song, or expressed my gratitude in another way. But I never took from Mama Cacao without leaving something in return.

When my basket was packed with yellow, red, orange, and tie-dyed yonic fruits, I knew I had harvested all I needed for this moon cycle. As I walked back home, I joined the others, and together, we built a large fire in honor of the abundant cacao harvest we had just been gifted. Throughout the following week, we tended to the seeds by fermenting, drying, toasting, peeling, and grinding them so that we could make artisanal ceremonial-grade chocolate. Once we prepared our chocolate with love, we gathered again in a circle around the fire.

A cacao ceremony is a beautiful way to honor the four elements of Earth, Air, Water, and Fire. The cacao beans themselves, a toasted and fermented preparation of the seeds of the cacao fruit, represent the Earth element. Each sacred seed carries the potential to birth an entirely new cacao tree. So, receiving these seeds in the form of heart medicine is no small thing.

The water poured into the giant pot and mixed with the cacao represents the Water element. Blending the cacao with water is essential so your internal waters and emotions may flow freely throughout the ceremony.

The large sacred fire where the cacao is brewed represents the Fire element. The fire supports your inner capacity to transform all you no longer need and send it to the creator in sacred smoke. The fire brings heat, warmth, and nourishment to your heart. The fire brings light to a dark night.

To honor the element of Air, we sing, dance, breathe, and allow our bodies to move freely with the wind.

Cacao medicine is wisely in tune with the melody of your heart. Whatever emotion is present in your heart while drinking this medicine will be brought to the light and perhaps intensified. If you feel some grief and sadness, the cacao may lead you to shed cleansing tears. If you feel grateful and ecstatic, you may feel deeper joy and connectedness after drinking cacao. If you feel anger and resentment in your heart, you may feel the cacao soften your edges and guide you into a dance of forgiveness. Let yourself be guided by the cacao medicine without resisting her true wisdom.

And trust in your own medicine working alongside the spirit of the cacao. You don't need to harvest the cacao and gather hundreds of humans for a potent cacao ceremony. You can even prepare yourself one intentional cup of hot chocolate and hold your ceremony as an act of self-love. Or you can share this cacao with a loved one or a few dear friends. Discover what you like to sprinkle into your cacao to give it the special touch of your essence. There is no wrong or right way to prepare cacao if your heart is open and your intentions are pure.

Traditionally, cacao is prepared with spice, a magical touch that you can add to your preparations to activate the cacao's medicine. You may want to add fresh ginger, turmeric, cinnamon, black pepper, or cayenne pepper for extra heat. You may want to add rose petals, cardamom, and a splash of vanilla for an additional feminine touch. You can create cacao as bitter or sweet as you would like. Traditionally, in ceremony, it is served with little to no sweetness, but sometimes, a spoonful of sugar helps the medicine go down! So, choose your favorite sweetener, agave, honey, maple syrup, or panela, and let your heart guide you in how sweet your cacao would like to be. You can try blending bananas, avocados, sesame paste, or coconut oil for extra creaminess. Perhaps you like to create different variations of cacao throughout your cycle. Lean into cacao as a reminder that several plant spirits will always be your allies and offer you their support.

Stories

The Pleasure of Penetration

Fall 2021 brings the winds of change to Northern California. My partner and I were making love, and I felt that co-creating such a healing and intentional sexual experience sometimes triggered memories of ways that sex has been the complete opposite of that in my past.

Far before I ever experienced penetrative sex, I had already begun to tell myself the story that my body was at the service of male pleasure. If I was attracted to a boy, I would start by denying my self-worth and tell myself that I was indeed too ugly, too fat, or too "not popular" to capture his interest. I would immediately compare myself to other girls, and to gain some points in this self-created and societally-imposed competition, I knew I could use my sexuality to my advantage. I justified that if he didn't like me for any other reason, at least he would like me because I gave him sexual pleasure.

From a young age, I have had a robust sexual curiosity. I often had sleepovers with my girlfriends, and we would make out and explore each other's bodies. My friends assured me it was simply practice for when we hooked up with boys, but I enjoyed sharing that intimate feminine pleasure space with them. Eventually, this whole situation of making out with my girlfriends caused some confusion within me.

One day, when we were having a sleepover, I asked my two friends if they wanted to practice kissing. They exchanged a glance as if there was something they needed to tell me. They felt I was taking "too much interest" in making out with them and thought I was a lesbian. At this time, I was probably ten years old, and while I did feel attracted to girls, I also felt a stronger attraction to boys. My friends assured me it was okay to be a lesbian, but they framed it in such a binary way that I felt I had to choose between liking boys or girls. I perceived that there was no neat category in which I could feel attraction to beings of all genders.

At my eleventh birthday party, one of my girlfriends and I began rolling around and acting out our version of a dramatic sex scene as we moaned and kissed each other, and all of my other friends watched. Suddenly, my mom walked in and demanded that we stop. She insisted we keep the door open for the rest of the party. I received clear messages that my sexual curiosity, especially toward girls, was something that I should hide or feel ashamed about.

So, I tended to lean toward boys. Even though I continued to explore sexuality with women throughout my life, it was only in my mid-twenties that I shared my first-ever intimate partnership with a woman. The pattern continued to unfold in which I felt safe and curious to open sexual containers with female bodies. Still, every time I found myself in a sexual encounter with a male body, I froze up, checked out, and became unable to speak my desires from a confident, sexy, empowered place.

With my first boyfriend, the first time I engaged in penetrative sex, and throughout our two-year relationship, I only ever felt two things during sex. Either I felt complete numbness and nothingness, or I felt pain like my body was utterly rejecting his penis entering me. Penetrative sex was never pleasurable, and at the time, I thought I didn't have the tools to navigate the challenges that came up for me around sex. So, I decided to endure this uncomfortable experience.

I came up with reasons to justify why I was okay with sex being something that happened to me instead of for me or with me. I felt I was lending my body as an act of love so the male body could experience pleasure. I never knew I could have a say in co-creating a pleasurable experience.

In 2017, at age twenty-two, I had my first ever consensual and extremely pleasurable penetrative sex experience. I felt grief that it had taken me so many years to experience this and also gratitude that it occurred relatively early in my life, knowing that many humans may live their entire lives without ever experiencing the kind of sex that brings them into deep pleasure states. I couldn't believe that beforehand, this lover was so attentive to ensure that I was ready to feel him inside of me. Since he constantly checked in with me leading up to penetrative sex, I felt at ease, relaxed, and trusting as I invited him into my body. And then, as soon as he slipped inside, slowly and carefully, he checked in with me and asked me how that was.

I felt speechless. I had no idea how to respond. In my sexual history, no male had ever asked me how I wanted to be penetrated. When I said I was okay, he asked me to elaborate and request the depth that I desired, the pace that I desired, and honestly speak to all desires that were alive for me. I felt the inner walls of my vagina soften into this visitor, and for the first time, I listened to my womb and asked her what would feel good in the present moment.

Sex with this lover completely changed how I saw myself and how I related to the pleasure of penetrative sex. Together, we opened a door for deep healing within my womb space. After exploring sexy time with this magical human, I had never felt so sexually activated. I remember those few months being the most lubricated period of my life, pouring my sexual energy into writing erotic stories and sexy songs. I felt that my womb cried tears of joy and pleasure in this phase, which is why she was always wet. It was deeply emotional to shed pain stories while creating new pleasure memories simultaneously. In the period of connecting with this lover, I wrote my favorite juicy kinky song, "Let Me Pleasure You."

I had discovered an important key to unlocking deep sexual pleasure within my body. I needed a foundation of mutual trust and verbal consent to feel safe exploring infinite levels of embodied pleasure.

Returning to this present moment, when my partner and I decided to engage in penetrative sex, he came in slowly and didn't move his body. I felt his penis fill my vaginal canal and was hyper-aware of every sensation inside my vagina. In the stillness, my vagina began a dance that felt like micro orgasmic pulsations drawing energy upward and then intentionally releasing. She felt so alive, awake, and ready to explore pleasure. This body that had felt absolute numbness for so long showed up in an empowered, activated state, prepared to speak to her needs, make sexual requests, and be an equal player in this game of pleasure.

Below are the lyrics to "Let Me Pleasure You."

Let Me Pleasure You

We breathe in
Deeply this sensation
Of total closeness and surrender
To the escalating
Mutual pleasure
My lips
Dance across your face
Savouring your skin
Down your chin
Up your neck
Sinking my teeth right in
As I softly hum in your ear

And I completely dive in to you
Resting my breasts
On your beating chest
And pressing together
Our synchronized hearts
And I completely worship you
Worshiping me
In this temple that is my body
Let me pleasure you
Tell me what you want me to do
Make me feel so good
Like you know I should
It's a feeling I can't describe
It's a warmness I can't hide
When I feel you
Inside
I want to run my fingers
Through your hair
Give you kisses
Everywhere
Feel the heat of your body
Against mine
Building up
I feel the pleasure
With our bodies
Intertwined
As I
Begin
To lose
My breath
It sends a shiver
Down my spine
Pull me closer
Exhale deeper

As I whisper
Let me pleasure you

Tender Hearts

I am full of gratitude, and there is nothing to do but celebrate this magic. As my heart giddily jumps for joy, I will share a detailed story of the creation of "Tender Hearts."

I had been in an intimate partnership for over one year. While we often navigated through turbulent waters in our relationship, I perceived we were in a stable, secure, grounded place. I felt that I could trust in the structure of our relationship enough to spend six weeks apart and then naturally flow back into each other's heart space. So I stayed home in my beautiful treehouse in a permaculture retreat center in Northern California while he went off to the East Coast for many adventures. One of these adventures included seeing his family. One of these adventures included going to Touch & Play, a queer, kinky, contact improvisation festival. One of these adventures included developing further romantic and sexual intimacy with a woman outside of the Touch & Play container.

Knowing that my partner was sharing tender, intimate sexual experiences with others gave me permission to explore. While he was away, I became curious about new ways to meet my needs and experiment with my desires. I noticed how often I perceived that I needed my partner when it was not him I longed for. I had just attached this person to a familiar road home that I could walk to meet certain needs. Sometimes, I felt a need for vulnerable, authentic, heartfelt conversation. Sometimes, I felt a need for playfulness and silliness. Sometimes, I felt a need for physical contact. Sometimes, I felt the desire to express my sexual energy.

Since my partner was on the other side of the country and mostly unavailable to communicate virtually, I searched for new routes and highways to fulfill these needs. I felt deeply held by my sisters in the community, by the wisdom of the cedars and pines, the chilly pond on the other side of my treehouse window, the Fall breeze blowing leaves softly back to kiss the soil, and the deepening of a new, unexpected friendship with Kinti.

Although he lived in a cabin directly across the pond, I would have called us distant, friendly neighbors at best for the first few months of sharing space in the community. There were many layers of judgments and stories that both of us projected onto each other in a way that created barriers for us to trust deeply in one another. Then, one day, the community gathered for a heart-sharing talking circle. We did our best to lay down our defenses and, using non-violent communication, spoke to what we were feeling and needing. It was powerful to look into Kinti's eyes from across the circle and, for a lingering breath, see each other's souls and hearts in the drawn-out pause between our exhales. As if we finally remembered that we are only here to love and support each other as we heal, holding each other for all that we are, which inevitably includes our wounding and shadows. It was essential to be witnessed and held by the rest of our community as we communicated, and eventually, both broke down in tears.

Once the circle concluded, we both looked relieved, as if a heaviness had been lifted, and we could soften into each other fully from our hearts for the first time. We hugged each other, apologized, and then he said, "Who knows, perhaps we have really beautiful medicine for each other that we have yet to explore."

This talking circle set a precedent for the blossoming of such an intimate friendship moving forward. At this time, he was navigating a breakup with a woman he loved deeply and searching for new ways to meet his intimate needs. So we naturally spiraled into each other's hearts and became each other's "number one in-person support person." We would share a morning-mate heart check-in ritual, which often included one of us shedding tears and the other holding space for the sadness, remorse, sorrow, confusion, and grief to move through. We were unconditionally supportive of each other during a potent medicine ceremony. We prepared delicious meals together. We would make each other laugh and bring lightness to each other's hearts. I felt that our hearts continuously expanded each day in an infinite blossoming of our capacity to feel love. I often felt so nourished by our interactions that this fulfillment would seep into my whole being throughout the day.

While we shared vulnerable space, there was resistance present in both of us to keep from surrendering fully to what was unfolding. He was grieving in love, unsure if he and his ex/current partner would continue to be in a lovership together. I felt a deep love for my partner. Still, it was challenging for me that my partner was off sharing all kinds of sexual energy with others and that he was making himself mostly unavailable to communicate, leaving me with all sorts of doubts and uncertainties about where his heart was. I felt his lack of care and consideration, so I chose to surrender to the mystery of the present unfolding.

I held space for the certainty that my expression of love for one human would never take away from or replace the love of another. I reached deep within the well of infinite love inside my heart, and I found myself completely open and ready to experience different forms of radical intimacy with beautiful humans who would all nourish me in unique ways. In turn, we would all show up for ourselves, our community, and this Earth as more whole and fulfilled versions of ourselves.

Our intimate love for each other: the fuel for our collective healing.

I felt deeply attracted to Kinti because he symbolized everything my partner was not. Of course, I know that comparison models aren't constructive since each soul carries their own unique medicine. Still, I couldn't help but notice the things that attracted me most about Kinti were qualities that my current partner lacked. I felt especially curious about these observations because I knew that how I felt about each of them simply reflected how I felt about certain parts of me.

Kinti had long, sleek, sexy dark hair that, in special moments, he let me braid.

My partner was balding and had frizzy red mad scientist hair shooting out the sides of his head.

Kinti had manifested himself a luxurious wood cabin home with a tea lounge, a kitchen, a tree growing through the center, a cozy bed, fuzzy sheep skins that he had tanned himself, two playful wild kittens, a warm wood-fired stove, a display of fancy hats, guitars, drums, charangos, plant medicines, and marigolds to adorn his temple.

My partner lived in a run-down crappy trailer with plastic bag windows, a door that wouldn't shut right, a lumpy mattress, and a pile of his dirty clothes to one side. I always found spiky plants and twigs in the cold bed, and there were often so many random misplaced items everywhere that I couldn't even find a place to put my bag down when I arrived.

Kinti had a successful career as a chef and formed part of a badass collective of sexy men who wove prayer and ritual into the culinary magic they created for their community.

My partner received unemployment for a while but couldn't continue because he couldn't get his paperwork together. Eventually, he picked up a part-time job milling wood.

Kinti taught me about Native American prayers, holding rituals, and working with different plant medicines.

My partner began exploring the medicine path through my guidance (and went to his first Peyote ceremony because Kinti invited him).

Kinti always looked his best, dressed as if preparing for ceremony. He valued sacred fashion, respected his body temple, and rocked intentional Earthy tones.

My partner's clothes were always dirty, ripped, and full of holes. His fashion style included genderqueer clothing that appeared to have come out of some dumpster or a musty bag tossed in some old farm storage shed. He would layer baggy green sweatpants with a flowy three-quarters denim on the bottom, and since the clothing never seemed to fit right, he would wrap this grandmother-style knitted scarf around his waist as a "belt." He would wear his current wife's grandmother's multicolor Mexican sweater that was once neon but now had collected so many layers of dust that it had faded into a mild rainbow. I often felt embarrassed, disgusted, and turned off by how my partner presented himself, his clothes, hair, and body. And I questioned what parts of my most wounded self matched him in that self-deprecating place.

So, without personalizing my attraction to Kinti specifically, I noticed how it felt in my body to feel called to rise and meet someone instead of sinking into my smallest self to meet my partner. As Kinti and I continued holding space for our tender hearts, when the time came for him to leave our home for a week of culinary missions, I noticed how quickly I felt dysregulated as I watched my fears of abandonment arise. I somehow felt attached to him, to the support we had given each other, and to the love we had shared. And I recognized that the kind of love I am calling in from the expression of my highest self is truly free of attachment. I am open to receiving sacred partnerships where we support each other to shine our light on this world, together or apart.

I noticed how important it was to voice my love and gratitude for him in my heart and the fear of not experiencing this love again. And just by naming these fears to myself, I felt much lighter because they seemed so sweet and silly, like the little girl in me not wanting the last day of summer camp to end, knowing that I would need to close a chapter that had brought me so much fulfillment. I wondered why this delicious warmth in my belly couldn't linger for a little longer.

Before he left, our community sat together in our wood-fired cedar sauna. Eventually, everyone had gotten out, and just Kinti and I remained. The fire had gotten low, and the sauna was pitch black. We had a medicine drum and sang our prayers with conviction as our voices and spirits freely shared a sacred dance. When we finished singing, I voiced some of the fears coming up for me and the deep gratitude and appreciation I felt for how we had so beautifully transformed our relationship.

He took in my words with deep humility and responded with loving authenticity that revealed the gratitude and admiration he was also experiencing. I reached out my hand, and we interlaced fingers as we brought our hands to each other's foreheads. We leaned into each other, holding hands in the dark, and placed our free hands on the back of each other's necks. There was so much love pouring straight from our crown and such a surrendered sense of safety as we breathed tenderness into each other. As we held each other I said, "*Te quiero mucho hermano*... I love you so much brother" And he responded, "*Yo tambien te quiero hermana*... I love you too, sister."

There was no way to deny that I had fallen in love.

But not with Kinti.

I had fallen in love with myself.

In many ways, remaining in my partnership depleted my self-worth and kept me feeling small. If you have read my stories to this point, it is clear that I haven't had the healthiest relationship with men. Yes, this partnership reflected my growth and was undoubtedly the healthiest romantic partnership I have ever had. Still, it was extremely unhealthy in many ways, and while I had evolved in a sense to arrive at a partnership with him, I knew that my personal growth journey could not stop there.

As I continued to open my heart with Kinti, how I saw myself radically transformed. I felt capable of manifesting abundance and fulfillment as I had never known. I began to wake up each morning with a desire to braid my hair and wear clothes and jewelry that would adorn my body temple, rising into the most radiant expression of my heart. During this phase of falling into more profound love with myself, I felt an endless stream of cosmic energy flowing through me with the potential to create, make beauty, pick flowers, and feel pleasure.

It's as if the creator had whispered a new breath of life within me, and I was taking in all the magic. I wondered just how long I could sustain this high and what were the limits of my heart in expansion.

Kinti and I found ourselves alone in the sauna a few weeks later. We had been inside for several hours, so the fire was burning low, and the small embers kept the space dark and warm. We played with each other's hands, slowly interlacing and untangling our fingers. I felt my heart pounding in my chest as my womb yearned to feel more of his body closer to mine. I was ovulating, and my sexual curiosity was more potent than ever. Until then, our relationship had never surpassed the limit of playfully flirty. Still, in this moment,

I felt a powerful desire to continue playing naked together, explore deeper intimacy levels, and co-create mutual pleasure. So I said, "I want to name that I am feeling really aroused."

Instantly, his muscles tensed. He pulled his hand away and became silent. I felt his nervous system go into panic mode as if he could not compute the words I had just spoken. I had no expectations attached to my desire. I simply felt curious to speak my truth and hoped that whatever was true for Kinti, he could speak it freely to me. After all, we had just spent a month cultivating deeply authentic, vulnerable trust in each other. But it seemed like I had opened an entirely different category, and he didn't know how to draw from the trust we had already developed in our friendship. Yes, we were in a hot sauna, but in those moments of silence, slight stutters, and nervous chuckles from Kinti as he searched for where to begin, we both began to sweat more than ever. Eventually, he said he needed some fresh air and asked if I would talk about this outside with him.

Somehow, somewhere along the way, something that had felt so good and joyful and pleasurable in my body, when expressed to Kinti, created tension in him and our dynamic. I was trying to express to my friend Kinti that this incredible thing was occurring within me. I've been waking up every day feeling alive, inspired, and full of juicy love, and I think our relationship has much to do with it. By expressing my arousal, I was potentially opening a possibility for us to continue expanding this beauty we were co-creating.

What if I had been met with that same excitement and curiosity when expressing my arousal?

Had I been met with curiosity, I would have felt safe to fully name my desires and dance in this juicy gray space. Instead, I felt that Kinti perceived the possibilities as a binary (madly in love or strictly platonic, romantic and sexual, or sister friend) when I was open to exploring new uncharted waters together that we could create to meet the needs of our unique relationship. Kinti went in many circles when talking outside, responding defensively and throwing his guard up. He affirmed that he found me beautiful but wasn't ready to explore any sexual intimacy with me right now. I felt him harden his heart to me at that moment. He ignored me entirely in the next few days, and our relationship had never felt more awkward.

So, as I often do in chaotic moments, I sat down with a pen and my journal. The emotions inside poured through me effortlessly as they transformed into words on paper. I was hurt that Kinti had been so willing to open his heart to me until I presented him with something that felt uncomfortable, and then he just shut the door to me. I know his sexual energy with women had created entanglements in his past, and he feared acting from a place of shame and guilt. But then I began to question if it was safe to bring all of me into our relationship or if only certain parts were allowed.

After I had poured my heart into writing and had given us a few days of profound awkwardness and breathing room, I asked if we could check in. I figured that sharing what I had written with him would be the best way to go. I felt there was a poetic quality to the words and that we could potentially transform them into the lyrics of a heartfelt song. Since, in the past, we had shared a beautiful musical connection, I asked him if he would be interested in co-creating this song with me as a comical relief to the winding medicine journey that has been our love. He seemed open to slowly transitioning back into our friendship but completely rejected the idea of coming out into the world with a cute song we had co-created about our tender hearts. I perceived that he was utterly embarrassed by the thought of publicly demonstrating our love through creative expression, and I felt his need to keep this whole thing secretive between us.

I felt disappointed and hurt because I visualized how beautiful our creative collaboration could be. I also felt celebration that he had given me his no. While this was a turn-off, it was also an affirmation that he was not ready to dive into this beautiful proposal with me. I thought, you can only lead the horse to the well, but you can't make him drink. So I knew that someday, I would be attracted to some musician and have these lyrics stored in my pocket, waiting to be birthed into a song.

Within one month, I packed everything up from my treehouse, ended my partnership, and bought a one-way ticket to Costa Rica to attend my mentor's Vocal Transformation Retreat. The whole group shared a cozy musical jam on the second night of the retreat. Slowly, everyone drifted off to bed while I and a talented guitarist lingered. I felt activated and energized, so I asked him if he wanted to improvise something. He laid down a structure of chords that could serve as a verse in a sexy drop D tuning, and then we flowed into a pre-chorus and chorus. And I sang Tender Hearts.

It flowed perfectly because I had memorized all the words but had yet to attach any melody. So, we naturally birthed this sweet song to feed the transformation of the dormant chrysalis into crushed butterflies in our tummies. I found deeply embodied joy in singing every note. This musical collaboration nourished me as he led me out of familiar patterns and guided me through new musical corridors. It spiraled into more profound beauty when we performed it with luring charango melodies and vocal harmonies. But the retreat was set to end, and we all made our way to different corners of the earth. And all that remained was the sweetness left on my tongue and the desire to stay open to new musical collaborations along the way.

One month later, in Lake Atitlan, I found myself dancing contact improvisation and making music with my newest crush. I asked if he would be willing to learn the chords of one of my songs so that I could sing along. Even though I get by with my guitar-playing skills, I mostly enjoy having my hands and whole body free to express my voice while someone else holds down the chords. He learned a handful of my songs and supported me in presenting my album at a live concert I hosted for my 27th birthday.

I felt so much pleasure and harmonious synchronicity while making music together. Knowing he would be leaving the lake soon, I asked him if he would be open to recording a video of us singing "Tender Hearts." Like capturing a screenshot of this moment in time of our creative connection. I am grateful for how safe I felt to continuously express my desires with him and know he could receive them. Early on, I communicated I felt attraction toward him and shared I was curious to play further. I gave him clear, juicy invitations, including exploring each other's naked bodies while lathering coconut oil onto our skin. And he communicated that he was most interested in exploring friendship, dance, and music together. We had different ideas about expressing our attraction toward each other, yet he never shied away from me. It took a lot of courage for me to speak my truth to him, and it took a lot of courage for him to continue showing up to co-create with me. We danced with divine cosmic energy and were free to transform this potential into infinitely any expression of our love. So, we channeled these emotions into a music video.

We spontaneously packed up our guitar, tripod, hula hoops, and matching hats and adventured to a private dock on the lake's shoreline.

The sun kissed our skin.

The waves crashed.

The wind tickled.

The volcanoes watched over.

The banana trees provided a small, shady refuge.

We sang.

We danced contact.

I played with my hula hoops.

We swam naked.

It was a perfect day in every sense of the word.

Interestingly, nothing explicitly romantic or sexual (not even a soft kiss on the lips) ever came from these crushes. A desire bubbled within me to continue deepening intimacy, and I perceived that it was not reciprocated in the same way.

So, I transmuted these tingles into deeper self-love and took pleasure in the limbo phase.

I enjoyed this warm feeling without becoming attached to any expected outcome of how this crush may evolve.

I trusted in the mystery.

I surrendered to the unknown of what will come next.

When I feel attracted to someone, I feel I am being continuously pulled into their orbit because I love how I feel in their presence. And maybe we discover that there's a shared mutual desire to increase these feelings of pleasure and connection together. Or since these sensations are alive in each of our bodies, we can feel them apart and channel them into our movement practice, dance compositions, writing erotic fantasies, juicy love songs, or any creative project.

I feel that having a crush is like having a creative muse. Some human comes along and inspires me to rise into my most radiant self. This light was already within me, but maybe some dust and cobwebs clouded my vision. Then suddenly, something comes alive, and I feel called to harmonize my room, cook my favorite meal, and spritz myself with rose essence.

This feeling of attraction toward another human can be expressed in infinite ways, and sometimes, we forget this by taking the crush so personally. If someone expresses their attraction toward you and you meet them with fear and resistance, there is little room for this love to expand into something that feels safe, healing, nourishing, and pleasurable for both beings. You are always free to claim your nos, mark your boundaries, and speak your truth. Radical intimacy is designed to meet the unique needs and desires of those playing the game. So, while the agreement may be less clear-cut than a "conventional cookie-cutter relationship," it is ultimately a pathway for deeper fulfillment.

Imagine your heart like a rubber band stretching infinitely in every direction. If you want to reach new uncharted lands of pleasure and intimate connections, you must also reach toward new lands of responsibility, accountability, and radical honesty. So, if you feel curious about exploring new kinds of intimacy with someone whom you hold dearly in your heart, may you have the courage to share what you fantasize about. Release any expectations about their response and be prepared to accept that they may or may not be open to exploring new depths of the ocean with you. And this is never a reflection of your worth. Even if you receive a no from this person, get curious about what the no means for both of you and how you can continue to express your love in a way that feels expansive, free, and healing. Expressing your desires to this person may be a step of embodied practice, affirming what you want for yourself and the universe. By claiming your desires, you create space to receive. Perhaps with this person. Or perhaps with another. Every step paves the way for your heart to fly a freer flight each day.

Thank you to all of the muses who have nourished my tender heart.

Tender Hearts

Please don't take it so personally when I say
that I have a crush.
It's really not about you.
Even though yeah, you kinda make me blush.
I just feel it flowing through.
It's the cosmic energy.
Opening up portals of radical intimacy.
Dressing up for the creator.
Making love to the divine.
Holding space for the purest light
Within me to shine.
Perhaps we'll feel this love
Together or apart.
Perhaps I will channel these emotions
Through my songs and through my art.
Oh be my muse.
Tender hearts.
May we tend to our tender hearts.
Oh won't you let me in
To the most tender parts.
And I will rest my lips on your heart.
May we have the courage
To share what we fantasize.
I'll hold you in your beauty
Thank you for holding me in mine.
Oh don't you realize
That we have the power.
To transmute everything into love
And now is the hour.
I don't know about tomorrow
And I don't know about yesterday.
But may we sink in deeper to the pleasure of today.
Right here.

Right now.
With these tender hearts.
May we tend to our tender hearts.
Oh won't you let me in
To the most tender parts.
And I will rest my lips on your heart.
May we continue to stretch
Our hearts infinitely.
Surrendering fully into our collective healing.
In this love there is no shame
There are no secrets
Nothing to hide.
Let us speak our truth
Breathe it all into the light.
I'm receiving all of you
And I am bringing all of me.
Refining the medicine
That we've been called to share so free.
Reclaiming the medicine of love
For all beings.
With these tender hearts.
May we tend to our tender hearts.
Oh won't you let me in
To the most tender parts.
And I will rest my lips on your heart.

El Llamado de la Selva, The Call of the Jungle

I arrived in Guatemala in January 2023, and my 90-day tourist visa ended in April. I felt a strong call to cross the border to Mexico and explore the jungle of Chiapas. Even though my parents were born in Mexico and I had been to Mexico City numerous times to visit family, I had yet to explore Mexico alone. Although I had never been to this part of Mexico, the waters began calling my soul. The songs of sacred waterfalls appeared in my dreams, luring me in, saying, "Come renew your spirit in our waters. Hear our melodies and share your voice with us. Come pray with us." I couldn't imagine a more nourishing way to get my passport stamped than to spend ten intimate days bathing in sacred waters in the heart of the Mexican jungle.

So, I began my journey to La Selva Lacanja, where the jungle engulfed me in her hot and sticky embrace. I arrived at the land of an indigenous Mayan family who rented out a small geodesic dome by a river that flowed through their land. I felt like a queen in my humble rustic jungle palace. I had come from many months of sharing intimate, crowded living quarters with many other community members. With this dome all to myself, lulled by the constant rush of the river, I felt the spaciousness expand my heart and enliven my being.

I knew I would call this dome home for a week, so I began weaving dream catchers, burning incense, lighting candles, hanging fathers, and picking flowers. I left little feminine touches around me and tended to the space as if I were designing and caring for my home. When I wasn't harmonizing the space, I spent most of my day in the water because of the heat and the mosquitos. So I played happily in waterfalls and creeks all day, like a fish returning home.

On the fourth day, I made plans to visit a sacred lagoon with the father of the indigenous family who was hosting me on their land. He typically dressed in traditional attire: a long white tunic for the men and a colorful floral tunic for the women. So when I found him in the morning dressed like a businessman with fancy pants and a collared shirt, I was surprised. He had forgotten that he had scheduled an important meeting in the morning, and we would have to delay our Laguna trip until the afternoon. It was interesting to observe how, as the day passed and he did not return, I began to feel like a little girl waiting for her dad to take her on an adventure. While I witnessed feelings of rejection and abandonment arise, I reminded myself that it did not reflect my worth. I felt disappointed that we had made an agreement, and then he let me down. Yet I remained centered and calm, enjoying my day by reading, writing, gathering wood, and building a cooking fire.

After my tenth river dip that day, I walked past some tables near the land's entrance and found a beautiful man playing the guitar. I felt my whole being smile because I had crossed him on the path the day before and exchanged a simple *"hola,"* with the extra kind of smile you sprinkle in when you feel attraction toward someone. I left that brief exchange yesterday thinking, "Who is this handsome man?" And here he was, making music at my doorstep.

We began chatting, and he passed me the guitar so I could share a song with him. He was from Mendoza, Argentina, making him the third Mendocino I had shared a brief and passionate shooting star romance. It only made sense to play him my original song about having a crush on an Argentinian guy. One of the lines says, *"deseo simplemente cebarnos unos mates...* I simply desire to share some mate with you."

Throughout the song, he looked back at me with loving eyes, in awe of witnessing my beauty, and I asked him if he would like some mate. He responded by saying something like he would love that but dismissed the possibility of it occurring. So when I told him that I had brought mate and my thermos was full of hot water, he smiled in disbelief that a beautiful gringa had arrived at this small nook in the jungle to share mate with him, mate that he hadn't drank in over a year and missed deeply. We shared a few delicious mates, savoring each sip and engaging in juicy, playful small talk. I blushed. He smiled. We both giggled as we felt the mutual attraction growing between us. He asked if I had any plans later in the evening, and I said no to the beat of my accelerated heart rate. So he asked if he could stop by later for some more mates and music, and I said yes. I told him to come over around sunset, the golden hour.

As soon as he left, despite many hours between our goodbye and our next rendezvous, I felt a joyful pre-date giddiness coursing through my veins like sweet honey. I made another cooking fire so my thermos would be full of hot water for more mates. I cooked arepas on the coals and made a fresh salad. I cleaned up the dome, lit incense and candles, picked fresh flowers, and played the guitar he had left me. I took another dip in the river and lathered my body in luscious cacao cardamom body butter. I put on a skirt and crop top with nothing else underneath and sat on my bed throne, admiring the scene unfolding.

I had manifested a sexy Argentinian musical mate-loving man, my spacious home full of sacred feminine touches, a river flowing at my doorstep, and all the birds and insects singing along. When he arrived, we shared some flirtatious chatter, and then he poured himself mate while listening to my songs in his private Aviva La Música concert. Each breath lingered sweetly in my throat as everything seemed to flow magically and effortlessly.

He began to share that he had dreamed we would meet each other and that I was coming to recharge his energy. I thoroughly resonated with dreaming and envisioning our future, so while I was happy to be a missing puzzle piece of his vision, I felt our exchange would also nourish me. Perhaps we could mutually charge up our energy. With a hopeful, childlike enthusiasm, I said that our energy is like a candle; if our light is shining, and we light another candle, this need not diminish our fire. We can keep multiplying our light. He smiled sweetly as if only this could be the case, but he insisted that in our exchange, he would take more from me, that I would give him more than he could give me. I found this sincere and authentic since he seemed to want to be clear on the energy exchange before diving deeper, and I appreciated the honesty.

Yet, it also felt icky to hear. Was I again stepping into a familiar pattern where I was the nurturer and healer to a wounded man? What would it take for me to rise and meet a lover who was full of gifts and medicine to nourish me in return? I also felt his comment was slightly self-deprecating, denying his self-worth and value. Who was he to judge how healing and nourishing this exchange would be for me? I shared my appreciation for his honesty but felt the gears of my mind churning in overdrive. Suddenly, this romantic bubble burst and spilled onto my lap.

I felt a need to reevaluate everything. Did I want to jump into spontaneous intimacy with someone who was more or less a self-proclaimed energetic vampire? Should I call the whole thing off and make love to myself? Yes, intimate love with another human being is messy, and here were my protective mechanisms and insatiable perfectionism kicking in and encouraging me to close the doors of my heart.

This reflection only lasted a few breaths of stillness, and in this pause, the mother of the land, whose dome I was renting, called my name and asked me to come outside. I was already a bit irritated in the back of my mind, wishing she would respect my space and leave me alone, but I stepped outside with a smile and asked, "*Que pasa*? What's going on?" *Qué pasa* is that she was kicking me out of the dome at night because they had accidentally double-booked, and they needed me to pack up and leave immediately. At first, I tried to calmly reason with her and explain that she couldn't just kick me out at this hour and throw me into the dark jungle.

I peeked into the warm dome, candles burning, incense filling the air, and decorations I had strung up all around, and

I felt protective of and attached to my palace. I felt insistent that they let me stay the night and that I could leave in the morning. But we only arrived at an agreement in which she offered a small cement closet-sized room I could sleep in for the night. So I walked back into the dome while this could-be-lover asked me what was happening. I began to roll around like a lunatic, blowing out the candles one by one and rambling to myself in playful disbelief, "Everything is coming crashing down... Aww, but I feel so at home... they can't do this. What's wrong with them?... I thought I had it all for such a brief moment... it's crumbling before me... thank you for being here... It's okay; I can let it go."

It was nourishing to play out this dramatic diva scene and be witnessed in compassion and love. I paused and asked him if he could place his hands on my back. I needed to take a few deep breaths and feel he had my back—such a simple way to ask for what I need and feel supported by touch. I still wasn't clear on what was unfolding within our dynamic, but I was sure glad to feel him breathing and laughing with me in the present moment. I told him we would have to say goodbye to this beautiful dome for a downgraded room. Regardless of the physical space, our spirits still wanted to be together.

So we transitioned to a tiny dark room full of dust, cobwebs, and dry leaves. It was an empty cement rectangle with a rundown, barren mattress tossed on the floor. "Nice window," he said, signaling to the black trash bag stuck on with duct tape to the wall. We laughed at how this was nothing like my feminine palace, but at least it was something. We lit a few candles, and the small fires brought a lovely ambiance to the dingy room.

Where were we before all of this madness? Well, I was questioning whether my heart was still in this. So I closed my eyes for a breath and began to draw my body near him.

I put my hands on his heart and drew my forehead near his. I felt safety, magnetism, attraction, tenderness, and care. My body said yes. He asked if I would be willing to rub his shoulders, so I straddled him from behind and slowly squeezed his shoulder, upper back, and arm muscles down to his fingertips. Eventually, I brought my lips near his neck without kissing him, simply allowing myself to share my warm breath with the tender space behind his ears. Then, as I began to kiss him, he turned toward me. We brought our torsos, hips, and noses near, and we slowly, lovingly began to caress each other. We lingered in the pause when our lips came near before finally kissing.

As we started kissing, I felt my body transition from, "Yes, yes, yes!!!" to "Woah, slow down…." I became very aware that this was the first human I was consensually sharing my sexual energy with since I had been assaulted a few months prior in Costa Rica. These were the first lips I had kissed outside my ex-partner's in over two years.

My mind had stories, and my body had emotions. I began to feel the nervousness in my accelerated heartbeat. I felt doubtful, fearful, and hesitant, and he immediately sensed the change by checking in with me. I celebrate how clearly I was able to ask for a pause and how truthful I was with the waves of emotions flowing through me. Some doubts and fears wanted to be seen and acknowledged so that I could continue to give a fully embodied yes to this exchange. I verbalized some of the needs arising, like my limits and boundaries being respected, and his loving response made me feel that much safer and held me in a tender embrace.

This, to me, is what healing looks like. It's not about pretending that the trauma does not exist in my womb anymore or denying my honest emotional response. It's about holding space for whatever arises as it arises, breathing through it, remembering how safe and empowered I am, and returning to the present moment.

I felt his body and soul entirely receptive to mine. He seemed to be in absolutely no rush to get anywhere. Instead, he just wanted to hold me in love. So we both took our tops off and gently caressed each other—our tender touch affirming that we were welcome to bring our whole selves. In a moment of a passionate hug in which I was straddling him, our beings held on tightly, and our breath became one. And then we heard a knock on the door, and the mother of the land was again calling my name.

We giggled and rolled our eyes like, what could it be now?! As we redressed and stepped outside, she explained that I could not stay in this room tonight and had to leave altogether. I felt betrayed after volunteering my time and energy to several projects on the land out of the goodness of my heart. That morning, I felt at home, then agreed to be relocated, and shortly after, I was asked to leave altogether. I went from feeling that I would recommend this beautiful place to all of my friends to feeling that I would never return to this place. I felt compassion knowing that these beings carried the rich wisdom of the jungle, having lived there their whole life but had no idea how to run a business or treat their guests. Finally, it became clear that I had to leave, and sexy Argentinian man offered that I come to his place. He had been renting a room near us for the last two months, and I was welcome to come over and spend the night.

When we arrived at his humble little room in a shared complex, the stench of dirty bathroom and sewage water was the first sensation to penetrate me. Then, I looked at the random items he had on the table. An empty Coca-Cola bottle, a condom, a pack of cigarettes, a broken shard of a hand mirror, Colgate toothpaste, and Raid spirals to burn away the mosquitos. Then I took in the sight of the lumpy, sunken mattress without a single sheet on it. There wasn't much of anything else in the room. I wondered where his clothes, backpack, or other belongings were.

Okay, not exactly a feminine palace, actually quite the opposite as things go. But I was grateful to have a place to spend the night and to be in good company. We made beautiful love, and then, in our hot and sweaty stickiness, we went down to the nearby creek. I took a dip there as he stood on the stream's edge like a cat afraid of the water. I couldn't believe he would turn down the opportunity to get in the refreshingly cool water. He couldn't believe I was crazy enough to get into the creek in the middle of the night.

We spent the next two days making endless love with pauses in between to cook by the fire and drink mate. It felt so beautiful to be seen in his loving reflection, as if it took someone from the outside to love and honor me for all of my imperfections, even the parts I felt most insecure about, to remember that I, too, can love all of me, just as I am. I couldn't believe how unbelievably aroused I felt in his presence. It was as if a rock had dammed the flow of sexual energy in my river, and as soon as the stone was removed, I felt like an exploding fire hydrant gushing with sexual desire.

So, after two intense days of co-creating mutual sexual pleasure, I was shocked when he did not want to have sex on the third night. He just wanted to cuddle. I felt rejected and disappointed as I sadly thought, "Cuddle? That's it?" It was interesting to observe how quickly my mind and body had made this interaction about sex when it was about sharing love and supporting each other's growth spirals. So, I worked on shifting my mindset, releasing what I thought the relationship should be so I could accept what it was in the present moment. Yet still, it was challenging for me to understand why he wouldn't want to continue diving deeper into pleasure with me, and he wasn't entirely communicative about why he wasn't feeling up to it. So my mind came up with this story that after two days of intense sex, maybe he just needed a rest and recharge, and indeed, on the fourth and final day of our rendezvous, we would make beautiful love. But on the fourth day, he related to me in a sweet, romantic way yet expressed no desire to connect sexually. I couldn't believe that on the last night we would share, he did not want to have sex.

While I felt disappointed, I transformed this into acceptance and surrender. The next morning, we shared our last mate and mangoes, but I was too nervous to enjoy the juicy fruit. I became aware of how intimate our exchange had been and how much trust I had developed in him and our relationship in such a short time. I felt uneasy about our goodbye since he seemed to be a ghost, and I thought I would probably never see or talk to him again. He had no material belongings. He carried nothing but the clothes on his back. He had no passport, phone, email, or social media. He refused to take a picture together. The only thing he could offer was the present moment. We kissed and hugged goodbye, affirming each other's beauty and thanking each other for the magic we co-created.

So then, about two weeks later, when my moon was set to come, she was late. Our protection method had been the pull-out method, but there had been one instance in which I felt that he cut it super close, and I questioned if any little spermies had stayed inside. I also knew that I was ovulating around the days we spent together because of my increased sexual desire, my vaginal lubrication, sticky clear egg whitey cervical fluids, increased physical energy, and the days of my cycle. However, I couldn't confirm the exact day of ovulation because I kept forgetting to keep my thermometer near me, and I hadn't been tracking my temperature. (I had been tracking my temperature diligently without missing a single day for over six months, and of course, the one time I was sexually active, I did not track my temperature!) So, I began to worry.

Every sign in my body told me that although my period was late, I was, in fact, premenstrual, not pregnant. Still, the fear of not being able to contact this man in the case of pregnancy felt like the worst generational karma playing itself out. I did not want my daughter to be born to an absent father. My womb sensed that there had been a visitor in her home, and through the sex and physical contact, a lot of emotions and memories had been shaken up and brought to the surface. My womb feared she had invited someone I couldn't count on to be there for me beyond the moment we shared. I think this is the only way I violated my boundaries in having sex with him. Going into our lovemaking, I felt safe and aroused, receiving a total yes from my body. I knew my boundaries would be respected whenever I needed to pause or stop altogether, and I felt that our intentions were loving and tender. But I knew he wouldn't support me until I shed him in my next bleed. We showed up naked and vulnerable in the heat of the moment, but now he couldn't show up for me when my period was late. Our energies are infinitely intertwined and will forever be. And especially from the moment of sex until I bled again, my womb was holding a lot of space for him.

I reminded myself that even though I couldn't count on him to show up in body or breath and couldn't reach him virtually, I could still communicate with his spirit. I decided to hold a ceremony where I would talk with his spirit and ask for his blessing to release my blood. I sat at my altar, lit candles, smudged myself with palo santo, and called upon the sacred tobacco medicine for guidance. Then I spoke my intentions, asking this man's spirit to accompany me. Instantly, I felt his warm hands on my back, and I got the chills. I was not alone. He somehow had a way of being in front of, behind, and inside me all at once.

He smiled and told me I was way too much in my head. Then, he told me, "*Vacía la mente y respiremos un ratito juntos…* Empty your mind, and let's breathe together for a little while." I couldn't believe how relieved and accompanied I felt by calling in his spirit and how receptive and willing to show up he was. He assured me that my intuition was correct. I was not pregnant because he could see my womb was not carrying a child. I felt tears and a breath of relief to affirm that I could count on him to be there, perhaps only in the spirit realm, and that although I would be a mother, now was not the time. After spending more time together, breathing, smiling, and crying, I felt I needed nothing more from him, so I thanked him and said goodbye. He assured me that I could call on him when I needed him. After this ceremony, I blew out the candles and went to the bathroom. There, I found the tiniest trickle of what seemed to be red blood coming from my womb. My moon had arrived.

Fantasizing About My Future Lover

After a long 14-hour journey through the winding Andean roads of Ecuador, I arrived at Vilcabamba, a place that I had lived twice before but hadn't returned to in over five years. While waves of newness instantly washed over me, the familiar scent of returning home permeated the air. The Andes looked as green and alive as ever, and even though the river was a walk from the plaza, I could already feel her powerfully rushing through my being.

As I put on my large *mochila*, backpack, and prepared to begin my journey up the mountain, I heard a sweet seductive saxophone melody luring me in. Hypnotized by the music, I was magnetically drawn straight toward this beautiful human with light brown skin the color of clay, striking turquoise eyes, and a cascade of long, thick, dark brown hair braided down his back. He had a hand-woven medicine bag strung over his shoulder, slightly swaying back and forth as he played. I listened in a trance as he gifted the plaza with his music. While many around were passively receiving his melodic medicine, I positioned myself directly in front of him, smiling, actively soaking in his beauty. He seemed so wholly immersed in the melodies he was channeling that he didn't notice my presence until he concluded the song, opened his eyes, and paused to take a breath. I felt drawn to say hello, as if some magical Spirit had said, "Go on, this is the human you have been praying for. Your soul is ready."

Trying not to get too lost in fantasy, I walked toward him and began chatting, introducing myself and thanking him for his beautiful music. As we spoke, I felt his entire body smile, almost taken aback by my presence, as if he, too, felt that some divine intervention was occurring in our having crossed paths at this particular moment.

He asked if I was also a musician, signaling to my charango I had recently acquired days ago. It felt fitting to begin my instrumental journey with a four-stringed ukulele, transition to a six-stringed guitar, and now embark on the journey of mastering the ten-stringed charango. I told him I dabbled a bit with string instruments, but I enjoyed singing most. I began humming a sensual tune, improvising freely on the spot, allowing my heart to guide my voice. And as I sang, he joined in perfect harmony, creating a vocal symphony with just our two voices and all of the angels watching over us with pleased, approving hearts. In just these first few moments of our exchange, I felt my heart had melted into a puddle deep into the earth, and magical love sparks fluttered around us like happy songbirds.

He asked if I would like to join him in the shade to share a papaya. I was delighted and in awe that I had already connected to this beautiful musician as soon as I arrived at this magical land. Now, on top of everything, he offered me papaya, one of my favorite fruits. We strolled together in a giddy state and sat under a large tree in the plaza's center as he pulled the fruit and a knife out of his backpack. Any relationship that begins by sharing abundant fruit is off to a good start.

He grabbed the papaya in his hands, and we locked eyes for a moment. He carefully penetrated the papaya with his knife vertically down the center, creating two perfect yoni-shaped fruits. He handed me one half, and I cradled this sacred fruit, flamingo color like the pinkish orange of a raw salmon's flesh, making love to the passionate red of a creamy cotton candy sunset. He placed his half papaya down and pulled two spoons from his backpack. I smirked at this synchronicity, almost as if he knew he would share this papaya with me, when he grabbed two spoons in the morning instead of one. We scooped out the shiny black seeds like small round pebbles and sent them straight back to the Earth surrounding the tree. Perhaps a papaya tree would blossom from this exchange. Then we dug our spoons straight into the honey-like flesh and took deep pleasure in the papaya, nourishing every cell in our being with her sweetness. Perhaps it was the love and magic swirling inside and around us, but we meant it when we agreed that we were eating from the most delicious, sweetest papaya we had ever known.

We began talking about our lives and how our journeys had led us to this present moment, and there seemed to be oddly striking similarities in our past and visions for the future. I listened with a smile and felt a sort of strange mystical twinkle in my eyes as if I was hearing myself share my vision but through the reflection of another. I felt almost speechless when he finished his share, wanting to shout, "This is my dream too! Yuju!" as I jumped to my feet for joy. But instead,

I lingered on one detail I felt most curious about. I asked him, "What kind of dance do you practice?"

He barely had to say contact improvisation before I could already feel it. But I let him say it anyway to play with that warm feeling of affirming the truth of my intuition. I responded with a sweet, *"Bailamos?"* as I extended my hand to him so that we may mutually help each other. I wanted to ask the universe what had taken so long for these two spirits who had been praying for each other to finally enter into a dance. I felt that our spirits recognized each other and we were dancing on the intimate grounds of an already-established relationship. But we needed no words. We let our bodies do the talking.

We began by bringing ourselves back to back, equally pouring our weight into each other, synchronizing our breath. I wondered if he could feel the back of my heart smiling. He was taller and larger than me, so it was pretty simple for me to slide my sacrum below his and lift him onto my back. We spiraled from here into a playful, energetic dance of lifts, twirls, and soft embraces.

Once our bodies were warm, sweaty, and exhausted, we ended up back on the Earth surrounding the tree. He had scooped me onto his knees with my belly to his belly. I curled my body into a C shape around his front, hugging his lower back. He placed his hands on my lower back, and we paused in this moment of stillness, returning to our synchronized breath. I felt so safe and comforted by his soul and body. I kept waiting at any given moment for his body to melt away and my alarm clock to ring, waking me up from this dream-like stupor. But as we continued breathing together, we grounded into each other. The fact that we kept returning to our breath made it all very real.

Eventually, I nestled out from our position, taking my time up as I noticed the proximity of my lips to his chest and neck. Without much thought, I decided to straddle him and bring our foreheads near. As we hugged, we pressed our chests into each other and felt the acceleration of our heartbeats. I became aware of my increasing desire to kiss him and lingered in that longing, savoring each sensation.

He delicately took my face into his hands and slowly caressed my cheek, neck, and lips with his fingers. He touched me with the care one would caress a small baby kitten. I nearly dissolved into an alternate state through his gentle touch, but I was brought back by this look in his eyes, signaling that he wanted to say something. Holding the back of my neck with both hands, he looked at me lovingly, through my eyes, into my soul, and asked me, "*Te puedo dar un beso?* Can I kiss you?" I responded with a fully embodied, yes, saying yes out loud and slowly leaning into him with a smile.

As we drew our lips closer and closer, we paused in the sliver between our skin and shared a breath. As much as we both wanted to kiss each other, there seemed to be no rush to get anywhere, taking pleasure in every step of the journey. When our skin finally touched, we stacked our top and bottom lips in an interwoven web. We shared soft, intentional pecks and created space between our lips to find each other's gaze. We smiled at each other as he looked upon me in awe and said, "*Hermosa*, beautiful."

We giggled at how quickly we had gotten so close, and I wiggled myself off his body into a standing. I exhaled a loud, audible sigh of pleasure and disbelief. I thought it would be a good idea to head up the mountain. Many hours had passed since my arrival, and soon, the sun would start to set. We thanked each other for this meeting and engaged in the formality of exchanging numbers when we knew that we would see each other again with or without technology's aid. If we had been brought together in this magical way in our first rendezvous, I began to imagine our future play dates.

I lost myself in a moment of fantasy, imagining us singing together, creating musical collaborations with our voices, charango, and saxophone, dancing naked by the river, and holding ceremonies together.

I returned to the present moment, picked up my *mochila* and charango, and said goodbye to my new lover for now. He sent me away with a delicate kiss on the cheek. If it weren't for the heavy backpack providing some grounding, I felt I could have just become a butterfly right then and there and fluttered up to the mountain's peak.

Below are the lyrics to a song I wrote upon arriving in Vilcabamba, reminding myself to sink into a deeper trust that my lover, partner, compañero, is making his way into my life in divine perfection when the space and timing are right and when our souls are truly ready.

Divine Perfection

It's been a long while I've been held in your embrace
It's been a long while my face met your face
My soul knows your soul, I've seen you before
I recognize your eyes, can you see yourself in mine?
Are you ready to be my reflection?
I surrender to divine perfection
 And in the meanwhile I'll keep my prayers strong
 And in the meanwhile I'll keep singing this song
 'Cause I trust, I know, I feel, I see
 That my lover is coming along
May our love be truthful and kind
May we share in generosity our body, spirit, and mind
What is the healing that we are meant to bring?
To each other, for this Earth, oh let it in
Will you remind me to see the light shining through?
The cracks in my heart when life gets too hard
Will you dance with me naked in the moonlight?

Sink into my skin, lift me up in flight
Will you listen to my stories with curiosity and ease?
Will you show up in consistency so together we may
weave?
All the medicine that we'll be
Our visions, our gardens, our dreams
And in the meanwhile I'll keep my prayers strong
    And in the meanwhile I'll keep singing this song
    'Cause I trust, I know, I feel, I see
    That my lover is coming along
With an altar of flowers
And peanut butter kisses
With deep belly laughter
Silence and stillness
With culinary magic
To harmonize my melody
With early morning waterfalls
Late night making love to me
With a land to build our home
Hands to seed and sow
Patience as we grow
Watching the river flow
With honey on our lips
Sun kissing our skin
Earth beneath our feet
Dancing in the wind
Are you ready to be my reflection?
I surrender to divine perfection
'Cause I trust, I know, I feel, I see
That my lover is coming along in divine perfection

Healing The Mother Wound: Kayari

After packing up my treehouse in California and closing up a year-long partnership, I was called to Costa Rica, where I sat in powerful ceremonies with sacred jungle medicine. I write this story to integrate this cosmic portal here on Earth. Before going into this ceremony, I was curious to connect deeper to the lineage in my womb, the stories of the past and future that ground me into the present moment. Knowing my mother was adopted, I always questioned the stories carried in my biological grandmother's womb. While my grandmother was alive, I had a beautiful relationship with her and could see how her stories and ways of being were imprinted in my mother. After all, she raised my mother, and nurture is a powerful force that shapes development. Yet, I always wondered about nature, about the bloodline that extended beyond my mother. What was my biological grandmother like? What about my biological grandfather? How would these informational gaps impact my relationship with the children I would bring to this Earth? In what ways could I connect to my grandmother through the spirit realm? Sitting with these reflections, I arrived with humility and curiosity to this medicine ceremony.

~

I am my grandmother birthing my mother.
I am my mother birthing me.
I am me, birthing my daughter Kayari.
Estamos todas juntas dando a luz.
We are all together, bringing light, birthing life onto this Earth.
I feel the deepest levels of orgasmic pleasure I never imagined were humanly possible. My womb is palpitating uncontrollably. The entire cosmic divinity flows through every cell in my body, and this pleasure is overwhelmingly uncomfortable.

Take a deep breath in, I remind myself.

Woah, please make this intensity stop.

I am going into labor right now.

I moan, plead, and pray that the being who comes through my sacred center is healthy and bathed in pure light. She says to me, "Hi, Mom. I believe in you. You can do this. You are almost there. I am choosing you to be my mother so we can walk on this Earth together."

I feel as if I am my mother.

I feel as if I am my daughter.

The contractions intensify, and I must scream. I feel the physical pain in my pelvic floor, the tears pouring down my cheeks, and the sweat dripping down my forehead. I collapse entirely into myself, a melted puddle of humility.

I cannot stop pushing.

A man supporting the ceremony approaches me and says, "Hey honey, drink some water."

I laugh at this suggestion because moving from my curled-up fetal position as a child within the womb to an upright position where I can sit up and drink water seems lifetimes away. I manage to hold the cup of water but can't bring it to my lips.

"Please drink some water. Just a little sip," he echoes lovingly. "Would you like to go outside and get fresh air?"

I can't move. How can anyone expect me to walk while I am in labor?

I begin the most sensual, arduous, slow, serpentine crawl toward the door, mustering the strength from the infinite well of energy within my being. The jaguar is with me. Together, we are strong.

I make it to the candle at the center of the room and feel exhausted and paralyzed. My body feels heavy, as if my entangled spiraling roots drew me deep into the belly of the mother's center.

"Here. I want you to drink some electrolytes. It's an Emergen-C drink," the medicine woman guiding our ceremony whispers into my ear.

"Emergency?" I question. It seems like an emergency, so I allow gratitude toward this woman to wash over my whole being. I trust her and will drink whatever she gives me in this vulnerable moment.

I try to take a sip and feel another big push coming. I give myself permission to let it out. I try to drink and then hold the water vessel to my heart.

This medicine woman is changing for me, for all beings present in this ceremony, and for the collective healing of all beings everywhere. As she takes a breath between her *ikaros*, her medicine songs, she whispers, "Drink it up."

Believe me, I am trying my best, I whimper and feel as if I am saying this to my mom.

The labor intensifies, and a handful of spirit angels guide me toward the door. I feel that I am pouring 500% of my body weight into them. Every step is an eternity.

"You are almost there. So close," he whispers to me as I whine.

The fresh air strikes me like the cooling breath of the creator, giving me a second wind. I can see the white mat I am being led to, and I feel so close to surrendering to Mother Earth, who holds me. I collapse onto the mat and look up at the sky. Just then, the clouds part to illuminate the starry night.

I feel held by the universal star spirits who watch over my daughter and me. They form perfect sacred geometry, and I know that Kayari is among them.

I get one deep breath in before the next wave of contractions snakes through.

May pregnant women give birth without pain.

My child is coming, and it almost feels orgasmic as I scream out harmonic cries, hum, shake, and surrender.

"It's okay. You can let it go. It's almost over," he assures me.

I am laughing at how unbelievably vulnerable it is to be witnessed by a man in this raw state. Yet, I feel his presence rooting for me, cheering me on, guiding me home.

"Thank you so much, Father," I say out loud.

He begins to sing an *ikaro*, and I chime in with my voice, my earthly anchor, throughout this otherworldly experience.

I hear people screaming all around me, and it makes so much sense. Women were meant to go into labor together, in community, in nature.

This is our rebirth. It is happening right now, and we all have everything we need.

I feel the spaciousness around me, and I spread my legs wide and throw them into the air in sweet surrender.

Just a few more pushes, screams, moans, and shakes.

"This is all happening because of sex," I think. "We were all created through the magical sacred act of sex."

The medicine woman comes over to me and gives me another blanket. She holds my hands to my heart and then brings them to my belly. I feel my womb pulsing intensely.

"Take a deep breath here," she says softly but firmly.

I begin to feel the slightest sliver of peace after the overwhelming chaos.

I know it is not over, but I feel the end is near.

I release a few last orgasmic pushes and sink deeper into the Earth, in disbelief that I can continue melting into the Great Mother of all life here on Earth. I erase the outline of my being and allow Pachamama to hold me and all of her children.

An angel comes to me and touches my belly. I open my eyes to see her smiling face.

She says, "Breathe with me. The breath is key."

As we take deep breaths together, I feel gratitude to all of the seen and unseen spirits holding me in this intimate birthing.

As I feel myself coming down from the mountain's peak, I slowly make my way back to the *maloka*, our sacred temple.

I sink back into my soft cushions where the ceremony started, and I begin to feel some autonomy over my breath and body. I put my hands on my belly, and then the tears pour from a well deep inside my cellular memory.

I went through labor, but where is my baby?

My grandmother gave up my mother for adoption and went through the entire pregnancy and birthing process to ultimately give her child away. In this shared grief experience, I felt more connected to my biological grandmother than ever.

As I cried, I heard the soft, sweet, innocent little voice of my daughter Kayari, and she said, "*Estoy aquí mamá, nos vemos pronto* — I am here, Mom, see you soon."

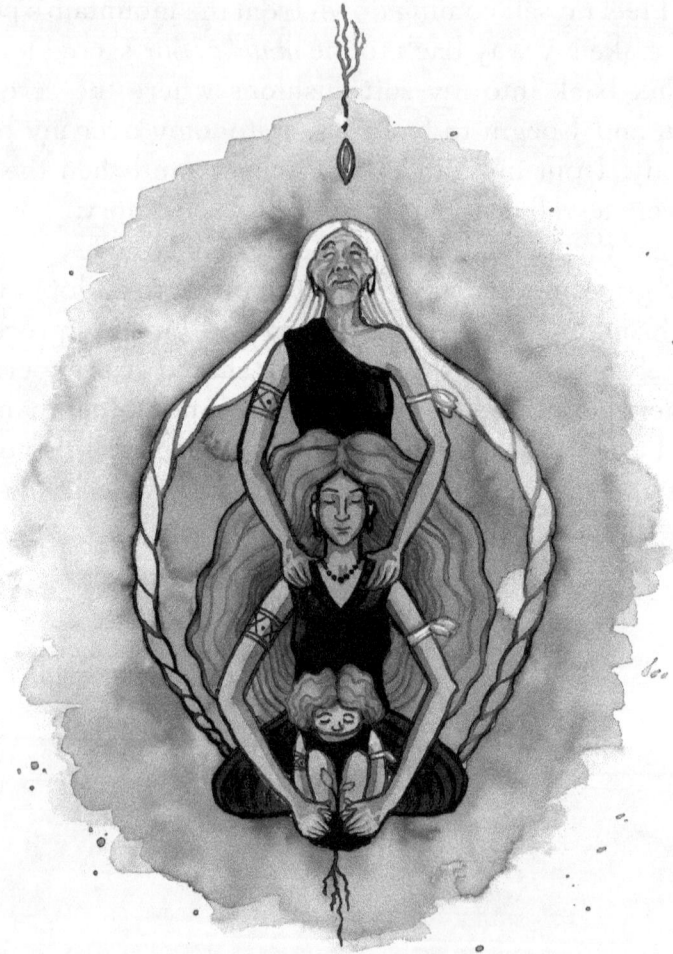

Lilith

Lilith, the farthest star from the sun, is often called the dark moon in our solar system. Legend has it that the two first humans whom God brought on to this Earth were Adam and Lilith, two equal humans in which neither one could be more or lesser than the other. Lilith was Adam's partner in the Garden of Eden. She felt unwilling to submit to him or grant him a dominant role. So, she decided to utter God's name three times, knowing that this would exile her from the garden and open a door toward her freedom. Because of her rebellious nature, she has often been demonized as a wild, uncontrolled, dangerous woman. And so this is when God took a piece of Adam's rib cage and created Eve, the perfect woman designed to serve man, a goddess with naive innocence.

Every human has a Lilith and an Eve within them. Wherever Venus appears on your astral birth chart, this is how you express your inner Eve. Eve and Venus are the desires that you can claim openly without shaming. It is how you connect to beauty and feel attraction in your conscious choices. Wherever Lilith appears on your chart, she represents the energy of your darkest, deepest desires that may feel taboo, that you may not express openly, that your subconscious seeks. You must take action to explore your inner Lilith, channel her dark desires, and bring them into the light. Eve is only half of the story of your desires, and to embody your full sensual spectrum, you must make space for the taboo to be seen and acknowledged.

This is a piece I have written to explore and liberate my Lilith.

What does your inner Lilith truly desire?

What is the story that she is longing to tell?

Lilith woke up to the sound of her alarm at 4:44 a.m. The hour of purification and clarity. With eyes closed, she quickly silenced the ring and began to glide her hand over her bedside table, searching for her thermometer. When she found it, she gripped it tiredly within her hands, with the soft slumber of sleep still embracing her like a warm blanket. She slowly pressed the button to turn her thermometer on and slipped it below her tongue. Thirty seconds later, her thermometer beeped and flashed 97.2. On day 16 of Lilith's menstrual cycle, her temperature still had not risen. She had noticed the sticky wetness augmenting significantly between her legs these last few days, the humid, moist fluids inside her growing alongside her ferocious desire to make love. She knew her temperature would rise in the next day or two, signaling that progesterone had risen and that she had already ovulated. But for now, her body was still ascending the fertility mountain, and she had not yet reached the peak of releasing her egg. As she connected to the pulsating fire within her womb, she felt her fertile energy buzzing an expansive light surrounding her and Eagle, who remained sleeping beside her. She slowly slipped out of the bed to not wake him from rest and walked lightly downstairs to the ritual room.

She lit four candles, one in each of the four directions, and sat on her meditation cushion in the center of the room. As she closed her eyes, she let the warm light of the candles envelop her in a soft glow. She tuned into the rhythm of her breath. "Tonight, Eagle and I will hold our love-making ritual," she thought.

Lilith and Eagle had been in partnership for several years and always prioritized exploring their sacred sexuality together in spacious, intentional containers. Making love together was an opportunity for each of them to cleanse themselves, ground, heal, and uplift each other through deep levels of embodied pleasure as they rooted and became one shared center. Lilith tried to put her thoughts about their love-making ritual aside to focus on her meditation, but she found herself getting distracted. Tuning into the life force energy of her ovulatory body gave her the desire to roar like a lion, moan, jump, and feel the strength in her muscles. She breathed into this potential energy and visualized a warm yellow fire growing within her solar plexus and filling each cell in her body with vital chi. She slipped into a trance, focusing on her breath and the sensation of the warm light enveloping her being.

By the time she brought herself back, the sun was beginning to rise, and she heard Eagle shuffling awake upstairs. She stood up and blew out three candles, lingering for a breath at the last lit candle. "Madre Tierra, Pachamama, Mother Earth, mother of all life on this Earth, on this day of my fertile window, I pray to you. I ask you to hear my prayers for motherhood. I trust in the mystery. I trust in divine perfection. And if it is meant to be, please allow Eagle's life force to catalyze the life force energy within me so that our love-making may be the portal for us to bring down our child from the stars onto this Earth through my womb." Lilith said her prayer in a low voice, summoning the Spirit of the Mother through the flickering candle flame, and then, with one fluid breath, she blew out the candle.

~

Eagle and Lilith began their ritual together at 4:44 p.m. Eagle ran warm water into the bathtub. Lilith harvested fresh lavender, calendula, and rose petals from the garden to sprinkle into their bath. When Lilith returned from the garden with a basket full of flowers, Eagle greeted her with warmth in his eyes. As if by looking at her, she could feel him saying, "Wow, I cannot believe that I get to make love to this beautiful woman." Lilith loved how easy it was for them to communicate without words. Sometimes, simply brushing each other's hands, squeezing each other's shoulders, or lingering for a few breaths of shared eye contact said more to them than limiting words could ever say.

"Hola mi amor, thank you for gathering flowers. The water's almost ready," Eagle said as he leaned into Lilith and kissed her forehead. Lilith pulled her shirt slowly over her head by crossing her arms and wiggling them up toward the sky as she swayed her hips side to side in a playful, seductive way. She repeated the same motion with her bra, slowly lifting it over her head and then tossing it onto the floor. With her chest and breasts fully exposed, Eagle could feel the warmth in his heart center growing to match hers. Goddess, she was radiant to him. Yes, he always found her attractive, but he never ceased to be amazed at how her glow changed in the days leading up to her ovulation. Her cheeks got redder, her skin brighter, her breasts more prominent. He wanted to embrace her in his arms and feel her warm skin against his. He also slipped off his shirt and wrapped his arms around Lilith, pulling her into a hug. Lilith leaned her ear on Eagle's heart and tried to match her breath to the rhythm of his steady beat.

Eagle's hands slid down Lilith's back and slowly made their way down to Lilith's skirt. As he hinted at a desire to slip her skirt off, he looked into her eyes as if to ask, "May I?" She responded by rocking her hips in a wiggle that helped him slide her skirt down to the floor. She then began to run her fingers along the skin of Eagle's abdomen, tracing the border between his upper and lower body marked by the outline of his pants. She slipped her fingers into his pants and slowly began unbuttoning them, pulling the zipper down as she looked deeply into Eagle's eyes with a focused, seductive gaze. Together, they slipped out of their bottoms until they were left standing naked together, embracing each other's bodies before submerging into the bath.

~

Lilith gathered the flowers from her basket and offered them to the water, blessing their bath with a cleaning, purifying, loving energy. Eagle turned the water off and grabbed Lilith's hand to lead her into their bath. As they stepped into the tub, they leaned their backs onto opposite sides to face each other and embrace each other's legs. Lilith grabbed onto Eagle's toned calves and began slowly massaging them. Eagle embraced Lilith's foot in his hands and began weaving his fingers into the spaces between her toes. Something was captivating about the way Lilith's feet could feel so feminine and soft, yet rough like a gardener, worn like a barefoot running wild child. Lilith began running her finger up Eagle's leg until arriving at his inner thigh. She felt a spark of desire pulse through her veins, pulling her closer to Eagle's chest. Eagle remained still, surrendering to Lilith's touch, and when she pulled herself closer to him and leaned her back into his chest, he welcomed her, embracing her in his arms. They took deep breaths together, noticing the rise and fall of their chest and belly. As petals floated around them, Eagle began to catch them and place them over Lilith's heart, forming a flower mandala between her breasts. He moved playfully and intentionally, picking one soft, wet petal at a time, slowly brushing her nipple, and then placing it on her skin. When Eagle was satisfied with his mandala, he brushed Lilith's hair back with both hands and revealed her bare neck. He leaned into her and began softly kissing her. Lilith moaned lightly, feeling the tides of pleasure beginning to turn within her body.

She reached for Eagle's hand and brought it to her face, where his fingers traced her cheeks, eyes, and nose. When his hands reached her lips, she let her jaw drop open, soft and relaxed, and slowly sucked one of his fingers into her wet mouth. As he began to pull out slowly, she gave him a soft nibble, trapping him inside her. She smiled at her mischievous bite and opened her mouth to free his finger. But when he had almost slipped out of her, she sucked him back in, and she repeated this motion of sucking him into her and then giving him space to slide out. She loved the sensation of his finger on her inner lips and tongue, the way that something so hard and stiff could enter such a soft place. Eventually, they both sighed audibly, slightly diffusing the sexual tension that was building. The kissing and the sucking took a pause. Lilith took space from Eagle's body, disentangling herself from his legs, and sat on her knees toward him. The bath had given her a flushed, rosy complexion, and she had a powerful glow in her eyes.

"Shall we get out of the bath, amor," Eagle asked Lilith. She nodded yes with a smile.

~

They made their way, naked, to the ritual room, where they began by calling in the directions. They stood together at the North gate, and Eagle opened this direction with a chant he accompanied on his medicine drum. He burned some cedar and smudged Lilith, clearing her with the sacred smoke. She passed the cedar smoke around Eagle's body, pausing at his heart. Together, they made their way over to the East gate, where Lilith chanted a song for *Águila y Condor* with her shaker and Eagle accompanied with his flute. Lilith burnt tobacco, and once again, they cleaned themselves with the smoke of their prayers and intentions in ascension as they made their way together to the third candle. Here, Eagle called upon the South by picking up his guitar and singing one of his and Lilith's favorite songs to harmonize.

"Gran espíritu, gran abuelo, gran abuela
Como soy me presento ante ti
Como soy te pido bendiciones
Y agradezco el corazón que has puesto en mi
Cuando vengo, ya sabrás a lo que vengo
A entregar mi corazon,
Corazon es lo unico que tengo
Great Spirit, Grandfather, Grandmother
As I am, I present myself to you
As I am, I ask you for blessings
And I am grateful for the heart that you have placed in me
When I come, you already know why I have come
To give you my heart
My heart is the only thing I have."

At the South gate, they burned sweetgrass and then made their way to the fourth candle. Here, Lilith lit the candle and opened the West gate with a powerful acapella chant and burnt white sage. Eagle and Lilith looked around the room to the four directions and smelled the dance of sacred smokes making love. Together, they called upon the Great Spirit in the heavens, raising their hands toward the Father Sky, surrendering to the Great Mystery. They welcomed Pachamama, Earth Mother, by lowering their hands toward the ground and closing their invocation with the seventh and final direction, toward their hearts.

~

Lilith and Eagle each pulled a cushion toward the center of the room and sat cross-legged. Eagle brought his *tepi* and *hapé* with him and placed them between their naked bodies. While the sacred waters of the bath and the prayerful smoke had cleansed them, they felt called to ground deeper into the present moment, set clear intentions, and brush away all that no longer served them with the help of *abuelito tobacco*.

Eagle placed some *hapé* medicine, powdered tobacco mixed with ash and other sacred plants, into his right hand. Then he scooped half of the *hapé* into the opening in his bamboo *tepi* and brought it to Lilith's heart. "Abuelo tobacco, please help Lilith's heart to fully open in trust and surrender so that she may experience deep levels of love, connection, pleasure, and fulfillment." He then raised the *tepi* to Lilith's throat and said, *"Abuelo tobacco*, please help Lilith's throat to be open so she may be free to express her desires, speak her truth, mark clear boundaries, and share her voice medicine with all beings." He then raised the *tepi* to Lilith's third eye, resting in the space between her brows, and said, "Abuelo tobacco, help Lilith to see clearly, to trust more deeply in her intuition, to let go of all negative thought patterns, and to connect fully to spirit." Eagle then placed the *tepi* on Lilith's left shoulder and prayed for her feminine yin channels to open and then placed the *tepi* on Lilith's right shoulder, praying for her masculine yang channels to open.

Finally, Eagle paused in the center, making direct eye contact with Lilith. They took in two full, deep breaths together. On the third inhale, Lilith paused in stillness without releasing or drawing in more breath, and Eagle brought his body nearer to hers. They maintained eye contact as Eagle came into Lilith, placing one end of the *tepi* up her left nostril and the other end of the *tepi* in his mouth. He then exhaled a direct, clean blow, serving as a clear channel to deliver the tobacco medicine through Lilith's spirit and body.

Lilith instantly felt the tears pour from her eyes and the burn in the back of her head as the tobacco's spirit snaked through her. Eagle pulled the *tepi* out of her and charged it up with the other half of the *hapé* medicine. They took a few deep breaths together, and then Eagle penetrated Lilith's right side with another direct blow, starting slow and finally sending all the medicine into her with a powerful breath at the end.

He pulled the *tepi* out of her and snapped around her head, clearing the energetic space around her. He slowly placed his hands on her shoulders and brushed his fingers down to her fingertips. Lilith remained still, breathing through the medicine, trusting in Grandfather tobacco and the ceremony that Eagle held for her.

After some time had passed and Lilith felt grounded enough to return, she thanked Eagle and then applied *hapé* to him similarly, adding her magic touches. Once they had both been cleansed by the *hapé*, Lilith reached for the coconut oil.

Lilith placed the ceramic bowl of coconut oil between their bodies and added three magical drops of rose essential oil, three drops of ylang-ylang oil, and three drops of cardamom essential oil into the mix. She stirred their love potion nine times, dipping her fingers in, and warmed up the oil in her hands. She asked Eagle to lay down on his belly and placed her warm hands on his lower back. She straddled his pelvis and reached to his shoulders, slowly lathering the oil into his skin and working her weight into his muscles. With each knot she found, she sent waves of healing and relaxation into his body, holding space for him to surrender deeper into her touch and pour his weight thoroughly into the Earth below.

Lilith noticed how his toned muscles took on a radiant glow from the light of the candles and the shine of the oil. She massaged his back slowly, reminding them there was nowhere else to be, no end goal, no rush. Their only commitment to each other in this ritual was to show up in fully embodied presence and love each other. She poured her love into him as the Aquarius water bearer pours love from her vessel, and she visualized how the energy in Eagle's aura painted slowly shifting flower mandalas over his back. She felt connected to him, even when they weren't making love. Lilith had a way of feeling and sensing him like harmonious golden fibers weaving together to form a spider's web.

She wanted to feel her lips against his skin, so she slowly lowered her face toward his neck. She noticed how her hard nipples brushed against his back, and she began to rock her pelvis in slow waves back and forth, rubbing her breasts up and down his shoulder blades. She brought her mouth close to Eagle's ear and began slowly blowing warm breath into him. Meanwhile, she reached for his head and pulled his hair from the roots to the tips. Lilith felt Eagle's desire growing alongside hers as she heard him moan softly and gently move his hips with Lilith's rhythm. Lilith took Eagle's earlobe into her mouth, slowly sucking and softly nibbling him. When she released his ear, she traced her lips down his neck and covered him in slow, sensual kisses, playfully intermingling a few nibbles in between.

Eventually, the energy escalated, and Eagle sat up and turned over to face Lilith, who remained straddled on top of him. They brought their bellies near each other and took deep breaths together, connecting to the orange fire that burned in their sexual organs. They took one deep breath together and began sharing a breath of fire, which they inhaled and exhaled through their nose, drawing energy from their shared center up through their cosmic orbit. They each visualized how their energy was nourished from their root, traveling up their spine to their crown and cascading back down their front. Each had their connection to the infinite well of cosmic energy flowing through them. And together, they began to enter into a shared trance. Eagle visualized a large oak tree and imagined himself drawing up energy from his roots and then allowing this energy to fall into Lilith. Lilith visualized an intense red rose pulling water through her roots and washing over Eagle. They remained in this infinity breath visualization until, naturally, their breaths slowed, and they found each other's gaze. Eagle held on tighter to Lilith and used his strength and body weight to flip her onto her back.

Here, Eagle sat up, keeping his center straddled into Lilith's center, pouring his weight into her. He reached for the oil, warmed some in his hands, and placed them on her heart center. They mutually felt the heat and fire growing in Eagle's hands and Lilith's chest, like two radiant lights that shared firewood and sparks, together becoming brighter fires. Eagle took his time massaging Lilith's neck, shoulders, arms, and hands. He then took more oil in each of his hands and slowly massaged Lilith's belly and pelvis. When he could feel her completely relaxed, he slowly made his way up to her breasts with a soft featherlike touch, moving in gentle circles, brushing her skin, intentionally avoiding her nipple, escalating desire.

Lilith rocked her body in slow waves synchronized with her breath, sending the pleasure from her heart center through her entire body. When Eagle finally began softly pinching Lilith's nipples, she moaned as she felt the pleasure and pain awakening her senses, sending a rush of euphoria through her whole being. Lilith continued snaking her body, drawing the sexual energy up, up, up through her crown.

Eagle's lips slowly made their way to Lilith's breasts, where he covered her in soft kisses. He allowed the tip of his nose to brush the mountains and valleys on her chest and gently began to nibble the tip of her nipple. Lilith remained focused on her breath and surrendered to Eagle giving her pleasure. Eagle made his way down Lilith's body, tracing her skin with lips and tongue, kissing and lingering on her lower belly. He continued to work his way down to her legs and teased her by licking the sensitive skin between her thighs. Eagle felt the power of Lilith's yoni opening between her legs like a lotus flower, and a strong magnetic pull led his lips to her outer lips. Savoring the taste of her petals, he began to massage her in slow circles. He noticed the way blood began to flow to her vulva and slowly began to spiral his tongue on the center of her clitoris while he continued to stimulate her with his hands.

Eagle drank her up, savoring in her flavor, like a kitten drinking abundantly from the well of life. He remained focused on his breath as he felt her breath quickening, her pleasure rising and falling like a wave.

Lilith felt her body melt into a sea of pleasure, riding the ebbs and flows like an electric current of life-force energy rushing through her. She remained in this trance of receiving pleasure for an immeasurable amount of time. Simply surrendering to Eagle, receiving his love, trusting in his medicine. Eventually, a large wave of desire began to snake through her, and she felt her body prepare to shake and tremble. She wasn't yet ready to orgasm. So she took a deep breath and drew this energy toward her crown as she reached for Eagle and pulled his body up to meet her.

Lilith brought Eagle's forehead to rest on her own, and they breathed heavily together, intending to ground the escalating mutual pleasure growing like a blazing fire within them. She slowly brought her lips to meet his and devoured the taste of her fertile juices like the salty sea rocking them gently as they made love. She took a deep breath as she became increasingly aware of Eagle's wand of light rubbing against her clitoris.

Suddenly, Lilith released a savage roar and flipped Eagle over onto his back as she climbed on top of him. She moved like a fierce feline overcome by the spirit of the jaguar, instinctually following her prey. As she swiftly rocked her body over his, she began sucking on his neck and covering his torso in her bites. She wanted to taste him, feel his scent inside of her. She dug her jaguar fangs into his flesh and scratched her claws down his arms.

Eagle felt the sensation of savage pleasure awakening every sensation on his skin. He couldn't help but moan through a gaping mouth as jaguar Lilith slowed her ferocity into soft licking all along his belly, inner thighs, and the sensitive space between his legs.

Lilith appreciated the calming of the jaguar within her, returning to a slower, intentional pace as she arrived at Eagle's lingham. As she embraced such a vulnerable part of him within her hands, she was overcome with such a gentle tenderness. She no longer yearned to hunt him; she simply wanted to nurture and lull him into a trance state, enveloping him in her love. She visualized a green light pouring from her heart chakra directly into him. She gave him all of her love without holding anything back. She licked and kissed him softly, maintaining his shaft stimulated yet almost surpassing sexual pleasure and simply arriving at unconditionally loving bliss. She loved him for all that he was. For the ways that he so gracefully embodied his masculine, creating space for her to rise into her most empowered feminine. They balanced each other like yin and yang, moon and sun, water and fire, air and earth, night and day. They complemented each other in their wholeness, without needing to complete each other, yet simply allowing each to shine brighter in their light through the love they shared.

She entered a rhythm of slowly moving her mouth up and down his magical wand, filling her mouth with his light. She could feel him enjoying the touch, surrendering to it, without any rush to finish. As she continued stroking him, she once again felt a rush of desire flood her like a cleansing waterfall. She made her way up his body until she straddled his pelvis. She locked eyes with him as she pleasured herself with the tip of his expansive light.

"You are radiant, my love," Eagle said softly and directly to Lilith.

"I love you," Lilith responded in a sensual whisper. "I want to feel you inside of me. Are you ready to fly my Eagle and fill me with your light?" she asked in a playful, seductive tone.

Eagle responded with a full-body smile. Never had he wanted her more. He loved how she embodied her fire, her power, her striking clarity and confidence. The way she was simultaneously so delicate, fragile, raw, and vulnerable. His love for her at this moment filled him with a blaze akin to the sun's light. Suddenly, he became a golden tiger bathed in eternal light, holding Lilith tenderly as their naked bodies became drenched in sunlight. Eagle rolled on top of Lilith and observed her glow for a few breaths. He reached for more coconut oil and slowly stroked some onto himself while he lathered some oil into the inner walls of her eternal cave.

Eagle looked into Lilith's eyes and, in a serious tone, asked, "Do I have permission to enter the temple, my love?"

"*Bienvenido*, Welcome," she responded with a smile.

At this moment, Lilith felt her flower open to him, creating space in her cosmic portal she hadn't yet felt before. Yes, she had opened her yoni many times in her life, especially with Eagle. Yet this time, she felt a continuous blossoming, peeling back layers of separation, tearing down walls, opening her heart, letting her deepest wounds be seen, allowing her purest love to flow through her. Eagle slowly slid into her with a sensation of infinite spaciousness. He had penetrated her many times before. Yet this time, he felt the oneness of their bodies, minds, and spirits merging into one living, breathing organism.

As he slipped into her, he entered slowly and deeply, and then Lilith held on tightly to his butt cheeks and said, "Be still."

After hours of anticipation, Lilith was extremely sensitive to the sensation of Eagle filling her up. She wasn't ready to feel so much stimulation at once, and she tuned into the subtle sensations of pleasure within her vaginal canal. She loved how safe she felt to express her desires with Eagle, ask for pauses when needed, and freely express her whole self and her spectrum of emotions. She began to engage her vaginal walls in micro pulsations, pulling Eagle deeper into her. She felt like she was having mini orgasms as light waves of pleasure rippled outwardly like a stream rushing through their bodies.

Eagle appreciated Lilith's attention to the subtle sensations. He noticed how tempted he felt to enter her and begin thrusting. Yet the anticipation and the micro pulsations added to the escalating heat rising in their center. He trusted Lilith knew how to listen to her body's rhythms and set the pace. And he surrendered to her flow. After all, he was a guest in her temple.

Lilith eventually said, "I want you to thrust into me. One deep thrust and then eight shallow thrusts."

Together, they slipped into a meditation, counting to nine, the number of completion, symbolic of the nine months a baby spends within the womb. They had talked about creating a life together, and they could feel their child was preparing to come down from the stars. In the last few months, they had shared similar dreams and visions about their love coming together to bring life onto this Earth. They felt ready, and they knew that the moment was upon them. Lilith was in her most fertile ovulation window. Their souls and bodies had fully merged. Just then, the full moon's light rose through the window and bathed their bodies in a moonlight glow. Looking out the window, they could feel the moon's wholeness emanating her fertile energy to match Lilith's ovulating body.

Swept into the full moon's tide, they began thrusting with more passion, snaking their energy up through each other. Gasping, sweating, remembering to breathe, Eagle could feel the overwhelming pleasure growing inside of him. He was not ready to ejaculate, so he slowly pulled out of Lilith and drew his energy upward.

Lilith sat up, and this time, Eagle straddled himself around her. They kept drawing their energy upward, breathing together the intensity of their connection. They brushed the tips of their fingers along each other's hot and sticky skin like a cool, purifying breeze blowing over them. Then they poured more weight into their caresses as heavy, warm water pouring deep in through their muscles.

Lilith spiraled with momentum in one swift inhale and guided Eagle back onto his back. She straddled him, stacked her hips with his, and began moving in slow circles. She felt his wand of light glowing brighter than a thousand suns, and effortlessly, she lowered herself onto him. They entered a fluid state, rocking their bodies in unison as Lilith pleasured her clitoris.

And then Eagle and Lilith dissolved; their stories and identities were pushed to the side and became light. They entered a breath of fire pattern, and their energy flowed in one microcosmic orbit. They trembled, moaned, shook, and crashed in a giant tsunami, splashing life force energy straight into the great reef of life.

~

Eagle and Lilith returned to their bodies and lay beside each other in bed, catching their breath. With their interlaced fingers, through their hands, they continued to feel the refreshing waves of pleasure roll in and out of them like the ebb and flow of a shoreline.

Eagle sat up next to Lilith, lying with her face toward the stars. He placed one hand on her belly and one on her heart as he began to sing her a soft melody. At first, she simply listened and received his music medicine, but then she started to chime in with harmony. As he poured his love into her through his hands, their song, their touch, and their love-making became their prayer so that the portal they had created may ascend into the stars and bring down a spirit from the heavens onto this Earth through Lilith's fertile body.

Lilith sat up and reached for the palo santo. They took turns smudging and cleansing themselves from each other's energy. It was essential in their practice of becoming one to learn to disentangle themselves and to return each to their center after their love-making. They let the sacred smoke wash over them and then took turns blowing out the candles. When they had blown out the last candle, the full moon's light flooded into the room, and they shared a brief moment at the window looking out at her light. Eagle embraced Lilith in his arms, holding her close to his heart, and together, as they watched the moon, they could feel her winking back at them.

About Aviva

Aviva was born and raised in the San Fernando Valley of Los Angeles to Mexican Jewish parents. Upon graduating high school, she spent several years living abroad and formed a deep connection to South America. Through a journey of returning to honor her oneness with the Earth, she has lived on permaculture farms and sustainable communities with other like-minded medicine carriers and artists.

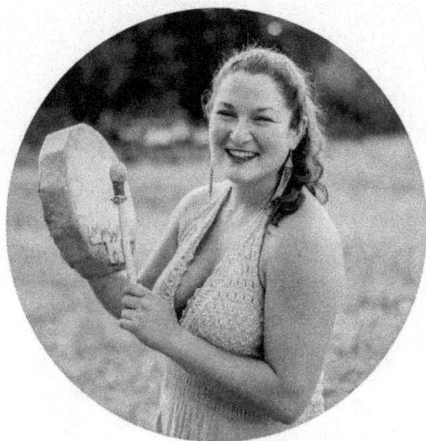

Aviva invites authentic sound and movement to flow through her being, channeling spirit as she dances and sings. She accompanies beings of all ages and genders to reconnect to their cycles through the medicine of creative expression.

Aviva is a songwriter, singer, and multi-instrumentalist; she has one album on Spotify in a musical duo called Las Parceritas Del Campo. Aviva is a dancer, constantly exploring spirals in her body movement, an eternal student and teacher of Contact Improvisation. Aviva's long-term vision is to caretake an abundant piece of land in the mountains for many moons, where the rivers flow, where trees and gardens thrive, where she can build her own cob home, and weave an inter-generational village with a loving community. *Moon Blood* and the *Moon Blood Journal: A Cyclical Mandala Calendar* are her first books.

Contact Aviva through cyclicalhealing.com.

www.ingramcontent.com/pod-product-compliance
Lightning Source LLC
Chambersburg PA
CBHW022049020426
42335CB00012B/612